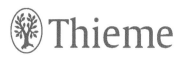

Botulinum Neurotoxin for Head and Neck Disorders

Second Edition

Andrew Blitzer, MD, DDS, FACS
Professor Emeritus of Otolaryngology–Head and Neck Surgery
Columbia University College of Physicians and Surgeons
Adjunct Professor of Neurology
Icahn School of Medicine at Mt. Sinai
Director, NY Center for Voice and Swallowing Disorders
Co-Founder and Director of Research, ADN International
New York, New York

Brian E. Benson, MD, FACS
Chairman
Department of Otolaryngology–Head and Neck Surgery
Hackensack Meridian School of Medicine
Hackensack, New Jersey

Diana N. Kirke, MBBS, MPhil, FRACS
Assistant Professor
Department of Otolaryngology–Head and Neck Surgery
Icahn School of Medicine at Mount Sinai
New York, New York

95 illustrations

Thieme
New York • Stuttgart • Delhi • Rio de Janeiro

Library of Congress Cataloging-in-Publication Data

Names: Blitzer, Andrew, editor. | Benson, Brian E., editor. | Kirke, Diana N., editor
Title: Botulinum neurotoxin for head and neck disorders / [edited by] Andrew Blitzer, Brian E. Benson, Diana N. Kirke.
Description: Second edition. | New York : Thieme, [2020] | Includes bibliographical references and index. | Summary: "Senior author Dr. Andrew Blitzer is an internationally renowned pioneer on the use of botulinum neurotoxin for functional disorders, with unparalleled expertise on this topic. Joined by co-editors Brian Benson and Diana Kirke, with multidisciplinary contributors, Botulinum Neurotoxin for Head and Neck Disorders Second Edition fills a gap in the medical literature. The unique textbook focuses on the use of botulinum neurotoxins for functional disorders of the head and neck, though with some aesthetic indications. The second edition reflects the latest advances and understanding of existing and emerging applications for botulinum neurotoxins, including new treatment paradigms, revised pharmacology, and an updated review of the literature in all chapters. Twenty superbly illustrated chapters cover the management of hyperfunctional, pain, and hypersecretory syndromes of the head and neck. Hyperfunctional motor disorders are discussed in chapters focused on blepharospasm, facial dystonia, Meige syndrome, oromandibular dystonia, spasmodic dysphonia (laryngeal dystonia), and cervical dystonia. Specific treatment approaches for pain are addressed in chapters on migraine and chronic daily tension headaches, temporomandibular disorders, and trigeminal neuralgia. The treatment of autonomic nervous system disorders is covered in chapters dedicated to Frey syndrome, facial hyperhydrosis, and sialorrhea"– Provided by publisher
Identifiers: LCCN 2019058275 (print) | LCCN 2019058276 (ebook) | ISBN 9781684200955 (hardcover) | ISBN 9781684200962 (ebook)
Subjects: MESH: Nervous System Diseases–drug therapy | Botulinum Toxins–therapeutic use | Neuromuscular Agents–therapeutic use | Head | Neck
Classification: LCC RL120.B66 (print) | LCC RL120.B66 (ebook) | NLM WL 140 | DDC 616.9/315–dc23.
LC record available at https://lccn.loc.gov/2019058275.
LC ebook record available at https://lccn.loc.gov/2019058276

Thieme Publishers Stuttgart
Rüdigerstrasse 14, 70469 Stuttgart, Germany
+49 [0]711 8931 421, customerservice@thieme.de

Thieme Publishers New York
333 Seventh Avenue, New York, NY 10001, USA
+1-800-782-3488, customerservice@thieme.com

Thieme Publishers Delhi
A-12, Second Floor, Sector-2, Noida-201301
Uttar Pradesh, India
+91 120 45 566 00, customerservice@thieme.in

Thieme Publishers Rio, Thieme Publicações Ltda.
Edifício Rodolpho de Paoli, 25º andar
Av. Nilo Peçanha, 50 – Sala 2508
Rio de Janeiro 20020-906 Brasil
+55 21 3172 2297 / +55 21 3172 1896

Anatomical illustrations: Markus Voll, Karl Wesker
Cover illustration: Ni-ka Ford; printed with permission from Mount Sinai Health System
Cover design: Thieme Publishing Group
Typesetting by DiTech Process Solutions Pvt. Ltd., India

Printed in the United States of America by King Printing Co., Inc.   5 4 3 2 1

ISBN 978-1-68420-095-5

Also available as an e-book:
eISBN 978-1-68420-096-2

Important note: Medicine is an ever-changing science undergoing continual development. Research and clinical experience are continually expanding our knowledge, inparticular our knowledge of proper treatment and drug therapy. Insofar as this book mentions any dosage or application, readers may rest assured that the authors, editors, and publishers have made every effort to ensure that such references are in accordance with **the state of knowledge at the time of production of the book.**

Nevertheless, this does not involve, imply, or express any guarantee or responsibility on the part of the publishers in respect to any dosage instructions and forms of applications stated in the book. **Every user is requested to examine carefully** the manufacturers' leaflets accompanying each drug and to check, if necessary in consultation with a physician or specialist, whether the dosage schedules mentioned therein or the contraindications stated by the manufacturers differ from the statements made in the present book. Such examination is particularly important with drugs that are either rarely used or have been newly released on the market. Every dosage schedule or every form of application used is entirely at the user's ownrisk and responsibility. The authors and publishers request every user to report to the publishers any discrepancies or inaccuracies noticed. If errors in this work are found after publication, errata will be posted at www.thieme.com on the product description page.

Some of the product names, patents, and registered designs referred to in this book are in fact registered trademarks or proprietary names even though specific reference to this fact is not always made in the text. Therefore, the appearance of a name without designation as proprietary is not to be construed as a representation by the publisher that it is in the public domain.

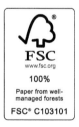

We jointly dedicate this second edition to our patients, whose persistent efforts to improve the function and quality of their lives constantly challenge, teach, and inspire us.

I additionally dedicate this book to my grandchildren: Jackson Blitzer, Samuel Wolkstein, Miles Wolkstein, and Ella Bea Blitzer.

–AB

I additionally dedicate this book to my parents Rus and Virginia Benson, my wife Amelia Gold, my mentors Arnold and Sandra Gold, and my supporters Jonathan and Maggie Seelig.

–BEB

I additionally dedicate this book to my parents Nick and Mary Kirke, my mentors both in the United States and in Australia, and finally to my husband Reade De Leacy and my daughter Delphine.

–DNK

Contents

Video Contents

Foreword

Botulinum neurotoxin is proving to be one of the most versatile therapies in all of medicine. Well known as a powerful poison, and still responsible for many deaths from botulism around the world each year, botulinum neurotoxin is very safe when used by a physician in carefully controlled circumstances. Ophthalmologist Alan B. Scott first identified the therapeutic potential of botulinum neurotoxin with his studies of strabismus, and since then the therapeutic areas have exploded. Because the toxin blocks neuromuscular junction transmission, the first (and still major) applications were for undesirable muscle spasms. Focal dystonias such as blepharospasm and hemifacial spasm were obvious targets and got early FDA approval. The senior editor of this book, Dr. Andrew Blitzer, is the pioneer who first used botulinum neurotoxin for the treatment of focal dystonia of the laryngeal muscles, spasmodic dysphonia. It turned out that facial wrinkles are due to contraction of small muscles in the skin (who knew that, other than dermatologists?), and that these spasms could be eradicated with botulinum neurotoxin injections. Subsequently, it became clear that botulinum neurotoxin could also block release of other neurotransmitters, and hence could be useful in autonomic disorders such as hyperhidrosis and pain disorders such as migraine headache. The indications are still expanding.

The indications are so broad that most specialists are turning to its use for conditions within their own specialty. Ophthalmologists, otolaryngologists–head and neck surgeons, facial plastic surgeons, neurologists, physiatrists, dermatologists, urologists, gastroenterologists, and rheumatologists now find botulinum neurotoxin therapy valuable. As with any therapy, it must be done right to be done successfully. Failures and side effects are often due to poor technique. Therefore, practitioners should learn to do the injections properly. There are various forums for this such as courses, but it is always nice to have a book such as this handy.

This book emphasizes the use of botulinum neurotoxin injection for those indications in the head and neck. Conditions range from laryngeal dystonia to facial wrinkles (otolaryngology to dermatology), from palatal tremor to migraine headache (rare to common). It is valuable for any practitioner using botulinum neurotoxin to at least be aware of all the possible uses. Since toxin should not be given more than every three months (at least with current guidelines), patients should not be treated, say, for their blepharospasm on one occasion and their facial wrinkles two weeks later. One physician comfortable with treatment of both conditions might do both in the same sitting.

This how-to-do-it book is supplemented with videos of the various techniques. A picture is worth a thousand words, and a video is worth a million words. This type of instruction is very valuable. People are good at imitation (now demonstrated to be due, at least in part, to the highly efficient mirror neuron system in the brain). Therefore, this text-plus-video can be an important aid to learn and/or to improve technique.

There are no better guides to botulinum neurotoxin therapy around the head and neck than Dr. Blitzer and his co-editors and contributors. Not only was Dr. Blitzer a pioneer, but he has about as much experience as anyone alive for many of these indications. This revised second edition has been brought up to date with advances in the years since the first edition had been published. For example, the chapters on oromandibular dystonia and temporomandibular disorders have been expanded to incorporate nearly 30 years of experience with these disorders. Additionally, there is a new chapter on the use of toxin for post-radiation therapy muscle spasm and pain.

This book should be valuable and readily available for anyone using botulinum neurotoxin for any indication in the head and neck region.

Mark Hallett, MD, DrMed(Hon)
Chief, Human Motor Control Section
National Institute of Neurological Disorders and Stroke
National Institutes of Health
Bethesda, Maryland

Foreword

In the current environment of instant access to the latest medical advances in most fields, the question could be asked: is there still a place for texts that some would consider outdated the moment they are published? My belief is yes, in selected instances. This second edition of the text on the use of botulinum toxin in the head and neck is a tour de force. Edited by the leading clinical expert in the field worldwide, it provides a career lineage to the topic that is unsurpassed. The wheat is separated from the chaff. Guidelines are presented as well as data that will serve as references by which to judge new information.

The full range of applicable sites are covered in print, detailing the specifics of dose and injection points. Videos detail the nuances of technique. The latter give physicians the best opportunity to get favorable results while mitigating the potential for adverse events. This text takes a single topic and explores it in depth. The breadth of information is singular. It is a must-read book, recommended for any student or practitioner with an interest in the topic. It is the magnum opus in the field.

Marshall Strome, MD, MS, FACS
Professor and Chairman Emeritus
Cleveland Clinic Head and Neck Institute
Cleveland, Ohio
Director, Center for Head and Neck Oncology
Roosevelt St. Luke's Hospital
New York, New York

Preface

This book fills the gap in the medical literature that had existed about management techniques using botulinum neurotoxins for hyperfunctional, hypersecretory, and pain syndromes of the head and neck. This updated second edition addresses the motor, sensory, and autonomic nervous system; reviews the pharmacology of botulinum neurotoxins; and discusses the indications and techniques for their use. Each section is linked to a video of the injection for that indication. The hyperfunctional motor disorders are discussed in several chapters that address blepharospasm, facial dystonia, Meige syndrome, oromandibular dystonia, spasmodic dysphonia (laryngeal dystonia), and cervical dystonia. The chapters review the diagnosis and phenomenology of these disorders and discuss the approaches to using toxin therapy in the different muscles. Other hyperfunctional disorders reviewed in this volume include hemifacial spasm, facial lines and wrinkles, upper and lower esophageal sphincter spasm, and palatal myoclonus. Several chapters discuss the effects of toxin on the afferent nervous system and pain syndromes. The effects of toxin on the release of peripheral pain mediators and the consequent change in the central pain thresholds are reviewed. Specific treatment approaches for pain are addressed in chapters on migraine and chronic daily tension headaches, temporomandibular disorders, trigeminal neuralgia, and radiation induced spasm and pain. Management of autonomic nervous system disorders is also reviewed and specific management of autonomic disorders such as Frey syndrome, facial hyperhydrosis, and sialorrhea is discussed.

This second edition should be of value for clinicians who provide care to patients with hyperfunctional motor disorders, pain and sensory disorders, and secretory disorders of the head and neck. These clinicians include otolaryngologists–head and neck surgeons, neurologists, dentists, dermatologists, pain specialists, physical medicine and rehabilitation specialists and all others who may treat these disorders as well as students. The book can serve as a guide to using botulinum neurotoxins therapeutically to treat patients with motor, sensory and autonomic nervous system disorders of the head and neck.

Acknowledgments

We thank all of our contributors for sharing their expertise with the readers of this book. We thank the editorial staff at Thieme Medical Publishers for their advice, effort, and encouragement throughout the writing and editorial process. We also thank Peter Morgen Blitzer for his filming, editing, and production of the accompanying videos.

Contributors

Ronda E. Alexander, MD, FACS
Assistant Professor of Otorhinolaryngology–Head and Neck Surgery
McGovern Medical School
University of Texas Health Science Center
Houston, Texas

Brian E. Benson, MD, FACS
Chairman
Department of Otolaryngology–Head and Neck Surgery
Hackensack Meridian School of Medicine
Hackensack, New Jersey

Boris L. Bentsianov, MD
Assistant Professor of Otolaryngology–Head and Neck Surgery
Director of Laryngology and Voice Disorders
SUNY Downstate Medical Center
Brooklyn, New York

William J. Binder, MD, FACS
Assistant Clinical Professor
Department of Head and Neck Surgery
UCLA School of Medicine
Los Angeles, California

Muna I. Bitar, PharmD
Associate Director in Medical Affairs
Regeneron Pharmaceuticals Inc.
West Caldwell, New Jersey

Andrew Blitzer, MD, DDS, FACS
Professor Emeritus of Otolaryngology–Head and Neck Surgery
Columbia University College of Physicians and Surgeons
Adjunct Professor of Neurology
Icahn School of Medicine at Mt. Sinai
Director, NY Center for Voice and Swallowing Disorders
Co-Founder and Director of Research, ADN International
New York, New York

Lesley French Childs, MD
Assistant Professor
Laryngology, Neurolaryngology, and Professional Voice
Associate Medical Director, Clinical Center for Voice Care
Department of Otolaryngology–Head and Neck Surgery
University of Texas Southwestern Medical Center
Dallas, Texas

Ajay E. Chitkara, MD
Clinical Assistant Professor
Department of Surgery
Stony Brook University Hospital
Stony Brook, New York
ENT and Allergy Associates
Port Jefferson, New York

Brianna K. Crawley, MD
Associate Professor
Loma Linda Voice and Swallowing Center
Department of Otolaryngology–Head and Neck Surgery
Loma Linda University
Loma Linda, California

Scott R. Gibbs, MD
Chief, Division of Otolaryngology
Associate Professor
Marshall University School of Medicine
Huntington, West Virginia

Elizabeth Guardiani, MD
Assistant Professor of Otorhinolaryngology–Head and Neck Surgery
University of Maryland School of Medicine
Baltimore, Maryland

Joel Guss, MD
Department of Head and Neck Surgery
Kaiser Permanente
Walnut Creek, California

Rachel Kaye, MD
Department of Otolaryngology
Rutgers New Jersey Medical School
Newark, New Jersey

Diana N. Kirke, MBBS, MPhil, FRACS
Assistant Professor
Department of Otolaryngology–Head and Neck Surgery
Icahn School of Medicine at Mount Sinai
New York, New York

Nikita Kohli, MD
Assistant Professor
Department of Surgery, Division of Otolaryngology
Yale University School of Medicine
Yale New Haven Hospital
New Haven, Connecticut

Michael Z. Lerner, MD
Assistant Professor
Department of Otolaryngology–Head and Neck Surgery
Albert Einstein College of Medicine
Bronx, New York

Tanya K. Meyer, MD
Associate Professor
Residency Program Director
Department of Otolaryngology–Head and Neck Surgery
University of Washington School of Medicine
Seattle, Washington

Niv Mor, MD
ENT at Summit
Division of Otolaryngology–Head and Neck Surgery
Overlook Medical Center
Summit, New Jersey

Daniel Novakovic, FRACS, MBBS, MPH
Associate Professor
Faculty of Medicine and Health, Central Clinical School
Director, Dr Liang Voice Program
University of Sydney
Sydney, Australia

Amit Patel, MD
Voice Center of Rhode Island
Warwick, Rhode Island

Scott M. Rickert, MD
Director, Pediatric Voice and Airway Center
Associate Director, Pediatric Otolaryngology
Assistant Professor
Department of Otolaryngology, Pediatrics, and Plastic Surgery
New York University Langone Medical Center
New York, New York

Maya M. Samman
Research Assistant
Center for Voice & Swallowing Disorders
New York, New York

Jerome S. Schwartz, MD, FACS
Volunteer Clinical Faculty–Otolaryngology
Georgetown University Medical Center
Washington, DC
Centers for Advanced ENT Care LLC
Chevy Chase, Maryland

Catherine F. Sinclair, BSc(Biomed), MBBS(Hons), FRACS, FACS
Associate Professor
Icahn School of Medicine at Mount Sinai
New York, New York

Phillip C. Song, MD
Chief, Division of Laryngology
Massachusetts Eye and Ear Infirmary
Assistant Professor
Department of Otolaryngology–Head and Neck Surgery
Harvard Medical School
Boston, Massachusetts

Lucian Sulica, MD
Sean Parker Professor of Laryngology
Director, The Sean Parker Institute for the Voice
Department of Otolaryngology–Head and Neck Surgery
Weill Cornell Medical College
New York, New York

Senja Tomovic, MD
Vice Chairman
Department of Otolaryngology
Hackensack Meridian School of Medicine
Seton Hall University
Nutley, New Jersey

Amy P. Wu, MD
Founder, Soho Otolaryngology PC
Clinical Assistant Professor of Otolaryngology
Hofstra/Northwell School of Medicine
New York, New York

Nwanmegha Young, MD
Yale University School of Medicine
New Haven, Connecticut

Craig H. Zalvan, MD, FACS
Chief of Otolaryngology and Medical Director
The Institute for Voice and Swallowing Disorders at Phelps Hospital
Sleepy Hollow, New York
Clinical Professor of Otolaryngology
New York Medical College
Valhalla, New York

1

Pharmacology of Botulinum Neurotoxins

Muna I. Bitar, Nikita Kohli, Maya M. Samman, and Andrew Blitzer

Summary

Botulinum neurotoxin (BoNT) is the most potent toxin, which acts to block the release of the neurotransmitter acetyl choline as well as other neurotransmitters such as calcitonin gene-related peptide, substance P, and glutamate. BoNT has been approved as a safe and effective therapeutic option for the management of many motor, sensory, and autonomic conditions. This chapter will review the biochemistry and mechanism of action of the neurotoxins, the mechanism of action, the pharmacokinetics, and the multiple clinical applications possible with these neurotoxins.

Keywords: botulinum neurotoxin, motor neurons, chronic pain, autonomic disorder, neurotransmitter, antinociceptive effects, sialorrhea, migraine headache, dystonia, trigeminal neuralgia

1.1 Introduction

Botulinum neurotoxin (BoNT) has been approved as a safe and effective therapeutic option for several clinical conditions. The common basis underlying all of the conditions amenable to treatment with BoNT is overactivity of neurotransmitter or neuropeptide release. The clinical efficacy of BoNT is based on the localized and highly specific, but reversible, disruption of the exocytotic mechanism within neurons, resulting in temporary inhibition of the release of neurotransmitters after injection into specific muscles or other tissues.

1.2 Subtypes of Botulinum Neurotoxin

Botulinum neurotoxins are synthesized by a variety of clostridial species, most notably *Clostridium botulinum*, but also including *C. baratii* (BoNT-F) and *C. butyricum* (BoNT-E), and *C. argentinese* (BoNTG).[1] Recently, non-Clostridial bacteria, *Weisella oryzae*, was also found to produce BoNT-A; however, further investigations are needed to define the biological role of this novel bacterial toxin.[1]

These bacteria synthesize several immunologically distinct neurotoxins classified as serotypes A through G with over 40 subtypes. A numerical notation has been introduced such that the subtypes are designated, BoNT-A1 and BoNT-A2 for example.[2] Epidemiologic studies and in vitro characterization show that only serotypes A, B, E, and F cause human botulism, whereas serotypes C and D are prevalent in bird and cattle botulisms.[3] Furthermore, three hybrid mosaic types have been described, including BoNT-CD, BoNT-DC, and BoNT-HA.[4] The latter was originally termed

"BoNT-H" but was later renamed based on amino acid and genomic sequence analysis, this being the first new BoNT serotype to be described in over 40 years.

1.3 Biochemistry of Botulinum Neurotoxin: Toxin Structure

The biologic activity of the neurotoxin is contained within a 150-kd protein commonly referred to as the core neurotoxin. In nature, a single 150-kd neurotoxin is incorporated into a molecular complex that varies in size based on the number of associated nontoxic proteins, which are classified as hemagglutinins or nonhemagglutinins.[5] The largest neurotoxin complex is 900-kd, formed only by the A serotype. Type A contains seven subtypes termed A1-A7 based on sequencing previously been described.[6] It remains unclear how these amino acid differences affect the subtype's biologic activity and only a few differences in characteristics have been elucidated. BoNT-A2 has been shown to enter cells faster than BoNT-A1,[7] to more potently inhibit the grip strength in rats after local administration, and to be more potent in the hemidiaphragm assay.[8,9]

Serotypes A, B, C1, and hemagglutinin-positive D are in the form of 500-kd and 300-kd complexes, whereas serotypes E, F, and hemagglutinin-negative D form only 300-kd complexes.[10] The neurotoxin complex is known to stabilize and protect the core neurotoxin against thermal and pH stress in addition to shielding the neurotoxin from enzymatic degradation.[11,12,13]

The core neurotoxin is synthesized as a 150-kd single-chain protein that must be cleaved or "nicked" by proteases to exert its activity.[14] Cleavage produces a di-chain molecule consisting of a 100-kd C-terminal heavy chain and a 50-kd N-terminal light chain metalloprotease that are held together by a disulfide bond. The C-terminal heavy chain can be divided into two domains: the N-terminal portion weighing 50 kDa is the translocation domain required for release into the cytosol and the C-terminal part is the receptor-binding domain that allows for the specific binding and endocytosis of BoNT into motor neurons (▶ Fig. 1.1).[4]

The tertiary structure of the di-chain protein is conserved through all clostridial neurotoxins; however, there is considerable heterogeneity between the protein sequences of the different serotypes (reportedly up to 70%), accounting for their different neuronal affinities, antigenicity, and intracellular targets.[15]

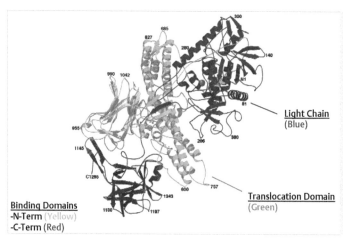

Fig. 1.1 Botulinum neurotoxin molecular structure. (Used with permission from Lacy DB, Tepp W, Cohen AC, et al. Crystal structure of botulinum neurotoxin type A and implication for toxicity. Nat Struct Biol 1998;5:898–902.)

Light Chain (Blue)

Translocation Domain (Green)

Binding Domains
-N-Term (Yellow)
-C-Term (Red)

1.4 Mechanism of Action

In the treatment of skeletal muscle over-activity, BoNTs inhibit acetylcholine release at the neuromuscular junction, thereby reducing excessive muscle contractions. This inhibition of calcium-dependent vesicular neurotransmitter release occurs via a multiple-step process. In the first step, the neurotoxin must dissociate from its protective protein shield to allow binding of the free neurotoxin to the neuronal surface. The kinetics of dissociation in vivo are currently unknown, but the stability of the neurotoxin complex is known to be affected by basic pH and increasing ionic strength of the solute.[16,17]

The binding of the free BoNT to the neuron is accomplished through the interaction of the heavy chain of the 150-kd neurotoxin with neuronal receptors that are located predominantly, but not exclusively, on cholinergic nerve terminals. For BoNT-A (the most commonly used in clinical practice), a two-receptor mechanism has been proposed: the neurotoxin first interacts with a cell-surface resident ganglioside that serves to retain the neurotoxin close to the plasma membrane, facilitating the binding of the neurotoxin with its cognate protein receptor. The protein receptor for type A, E, and F neurotoxins has been identified as SV2, a constituent protein of the synaptic vesicle.[18,19,20,21] The neurotoxin is only able to bind to SV2 when the protein is exposed on the cell surface during neurotransmitter release. Thus, the neurotoxin preferentially enters neurons that are actively secreting neurotransmitter or neuropeptides.[19] The receptor molecules for serotypes A and B are distinct, with the protein receptor for types B and G identified as another synaptic vesicle protein

known as synaptotagmin.[20] Other serotypes may also bind to unique sites, but they have not been characterized at this time.

After binding, BoNTs are internalized into the neuron via receptor-mediated endocytosis.[22] The neurotoxin undergoes a conformational change inside the acidified endocytotic vesicles, allowing the translocation domain to interact with the membrane of the endocytotic vesicle, providing a portal to enable the light chain to traverse the wall of the endosome.[23] The low pH in the endocytotic vesicle also reduces the disulfide bond, which releases the light chain from the heavy chain, freeing it to enter the neuronal cytosol.[24] Once inside the cytosol, the light chain, which contains a zinc-dependent endopeptidase, disrupts one or more of the SNARE (soluble N-ethylmaleimide-fusion-protein attachment protein receptor complex) proteins necessary for vesicle docking and fusion, thereby reducing exocytotic neurotransmitter release (▶ Fig. 1.2).[25]

Impairing the function of the SNARE complex causes inhibition of neurotransmission, leading to flaccid paralysis and potentially death. Each serotype cleaves a specific peptide bond on one or more of these proteins. Type A neurotoxin cleaves the membrane-associated SNARE protein SNAP-25 (synaptosomal-associated membrane protein weighing 25 kDa), whereas type B neurotoxin cleaves the vesicular-associated protein VAMP (synaptobrevin). It has been recently proposed that modulation of the interstitial zinc concentration might alter the clinical efficacy of BoNT activity; however, this concept remains unexplored currently. Of note, BoNT-HA cleaves VAMP-2, or synaptobrevin, which is identical to the behavior of BoNT-FA.[4]

1.5 Pharmacokinetics of Botulinum Neurotoxin

The relative duration of inhibition of neurotransmitter release varies among serotypes, presumably based on the half-life of the light-chain[26] and the time it has taken for the neuron to restore intact SNARE proteins (▶ Fig. 1.3). In a preclinical model, the duration of effect was the longest for type A, followed by types C1, B, F, and E.[27] Following injection in human muscles, serotypes A and C1 appear to have the longest duration of effect.[28]

The recovery of neuronal activity following BoNT-induced denervation has been examined in several preclinical models.[29,30,31] Early studies showed that axonal sprouts developed from the affected nerves, likely in response to growth factor secretion from the denervated muscle. These sprouts are active and produce temporary reinnervation during the early recovery phase. The exact duration of the pharmacologic action of BoNT in neurons is not known; however, during the later phase of recovery, vesicular release has been found to return at the original terminal, a process that is accompanied by retraction of the neuronal sprouts. This suggests a process of sprouting that is associated with reestablishment of activity over time in the originally affected nerve terminal.

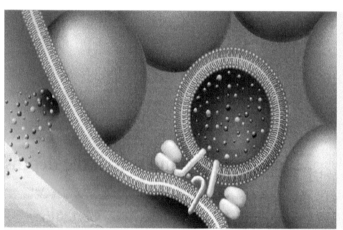

Fig. 1.2 Inhibition of exocytosis. (Used with permission from Martin TF, Stages of regulated exocytosis. Trends Cell Biol 1997;7(7):271–276.)

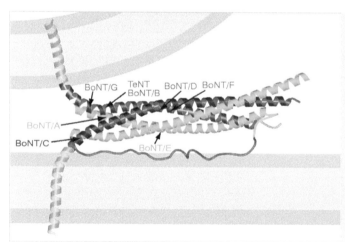

Fig. 1.3 Botulinum neurotoxin cleavage sites. TeNT, tetanus neurotoxin. (Used with permission from Sutton RB, Fasshauer D, Jahn R, Brunger AT. Crystal structure of a SNARE complex involved in synaptic exocytosis at 2.4 A resolution. Nature 1998;395:347–353.)

The inhibition of neurotransmitter release by BoNTs is reversible, which has both benefits and limitations in clinical use. The benefits include the flexibility to inject a given muscle based on its activity level, which may fluctuate over time, the avoidance of permanent interventions such as surgery, and the resolution of any unintended effects of BoNT treatment. The primary limitation associated with the reversibility of the effects of BoNT is the need for repeated injections; however, repeat treatment can result in sustained efficacy. As most conditions treated with BoNT are chronic in nature, a longer duration of effect is a desirable property and was the rationale for the development of type A over other serotypes of BoNT for clinical use.

1.6 Secondary Mechanism of Action

In addition to the inhibition of acetylcholine release from alpha motor neurons, BoNT-A also inhibits neurotransmitter release from gamma motor neurons innervating the intrafusal fibers of the muscle spindle.[32,33,34] The gamma motor system contributes to the setting of muscle tone and is known to play an important role in the maintenance of hyperactive muscle contractions in spasticity and dystonia. Reducing the gamma efferent influence in these conditions reduces the afferent feedback through type 1a afferent neurons, perhaps modifying, at a spinal level, the altered sensorimotor integration that occurs in these conditions.[35] At least some muscles of facial expression are reported to lack muscle spindles[36,37]; therefore, the contribution of this effect in the aesthetic applications of BoNT in the face is unclear.

1.7 Clinical Applications

Currently, the United States Food and Drug Administration (FDA) has approved two serotypes, A1 (Abo, ona, and incobotulinum toxin A) and B1 (rimabotulinum toxin B) for use in humans. BoNT-A1 is the predominant serotype of BoNT used for pharmaceutical applications and the best studied. Its potency, long duration of action, and localized activity in the inhibition of neuromuscular activity upon intramuscular injection have contributed to its use for clinical and aesthetic applications.[6] BoNT has been reported to be effective in managing hyperfunction of sweat glands (hyperhidrosis)[38] and salivary glands (sialorrhea),[39] in addition to other secretory conditions such as rhinitis[40] and gustatory sweating.[41] This suggests that injection of BoNT into appropriate tissues also has an effect on the activity of postganglionic neurons of the autonomic nervous system.[42] By blocking acetylcholine release in these fibers, glandular secretions may be reduced or blocked. In relative terms, BoNT-A appears to have a significantly longer duration of effect on autonomic neurons, with clinical benefit persisting as long as 6 to 9 months in disorders such as hyperhidrosis and overactive bladder in contrast to the 3 to 4 months typically observed for striated muscle.[38,43] This may reflect a difference in the recovery mechanisms in autonomically innervated versus somatically innervated tissue; for example, there is evidence that axonal sprouting does not occur to the same degree in the bladder following BoNT as it does in striated muscle[44]; however, other factors may also be involved.

Beyond the effects of BoNT on muscle tone and glandular secretions, BoNT-A has also been reported to reduce pain associated with cervical dystonia,[45] temporomandibular disorders,[46] and postherpetic[47] and trigeminal neuralgia.[48] Furthermore, recent data have demonstrated that one BoNT product, onabotulinumtoxinA, is effective in decreasing the frequency of headaches in patients with chronic migraine.[49] The mechanism of action of the neurotoxin in these conditions is unclear; however, it has been proposed that it occurs through the inhibition of release of neuropeptides and neurotransmitters from the peripheral terminals of afferent neurons.[50,51]

C-fiber nociceptive neurons are known to release glutamate and proinflammatory neuropeptides such as substance P and calcitonin gene-related peptide (CGRP) from their peripheral terminals in response to activation.[52] Release of substance P and CGRP results in vasodilation[53] and extravasation of other inflammatory mediators such as bradykinin, prostaglandins, histamine, and serotonin.[54] These inflammatory mediators either directly stimulate or sensitize peripheral nociceptors, triggering the sensation of pain and peripheral sensitization.[54] The sensitization of peripheral nociceptors may, in turn, trigger the release of more substance P and glutamate in the spinal cord, potentially leading to central sensitization, driving chronicity of pain.[55] Peripherally released glutamate is also believed to stimulate nociceptive neurons through activation of receptors on peripheral afferents.[56] SNARE proteins have been shown to mediate the release of these neuropeptides and neurotransmitters,[57] and thus the mechanism underlying the antinociceptive action of BoNT type A is thought to involve inhibition of release of these factors leading to a direct reduction of peripheral sensitization and, subsequently, an indirect reduction in central sensitization.

Newer data suggest a potential addition to the antinociceptive effects of BoNT. TRPV1 is an ion channel found on some sensory neurons that is activated by capsaicin, protons, and noxious heat, and is known to be upregulated in tissues during chronic pain and inflammation.[58] BoNT type A has been shown to reduce the expression of TRPV1 in several cell and tissues types, suggesting another mechanism by which BoNT can potentially reduce peripheral sensitization.[59,60,61] A-delta sensory fibers, which mediate acute pain signals, or A-beta fibers, which mediate touch and pressure sensation, do not release neuropeptides or transmitters from their peripheral terminals and are therefore not affected by BoNT. Thus, BoNT does not induce cutaneous anesthesia or interfere with the normal perception of acute pain.

1.8 Secondary Applications of Other Serotypes of Botulinum Neurotoxin

Kaji also developed a low-molecular-weight (150 kD) BoNT-A2 for clinical use from a highly purified protein derivative of infantile botulism. The first human study demonstrated the clinical efficacy to be 1.5 times that of onabotulinum toxin A with a faster time of onset and less spreading. Animal studies also demonstrate a higher potency to cleave SNAP25 than any other cell type as well as faster entry to cells. It may also be less immunogenic, but larger studies are necessary for confirmation.[62] Therapeutic uses of BoNT-A2 may include treatment for patients who have antibodies to A1 toxin.

Most recently, daxibotulinumtoxinA (RT002) is a novel protein composed of a 150-kDa BoNT-A molecule, with a proprietary peptide designed to be a long-lasting injectable neurotoxin with no animal-derived components or human albumin. This protein, which is produced by Revance Therapeutics, achieved the 6-month duration in two pivotal SAKURA Phase 3 clinical studies for the treatment of glabellar lines and delivered a statistically significant improvement as compared to placebo. A long-term trial assessing its safety is currently underway and pending successful completion; the company aims to apply for approval with the FDA and launch in 2020.[63]

1.9 Future Directions and Conclusion

The number of approved indications for BoNT has grown significantly since this agent was first proposed as a therapeutic tool in the 1970s, and many other potential uses have been reported in the literature. This can be attributed to its exquisite specificity: it is a single molecule with three domains responsible for specific functions including cell binding, translocation inside the cells, and cleave of intracellular substrate. Its biochemical properties allow for protein engineering and thus there have been approaches considered to enhance the toxin's capabilities or retarget its functions.[3] With a greater understanding of the pharmacology, it is conceivable that the range of clinical indications for BoNT will grow in the future.

BoNT has also been studied as a protein transporter given the potent and selective activity of BoNT on neuronal targets and its ability to deliver a 50-KDa protein domain into the neuronal cytosol. The highly specific heavy chain of BoNT has been used to target neuronal cells. Using BoNT heavy chain as a partner to DNA-binding protein may be useful not only for targeting motor neurons but also for utilizing BoNT's intracellular transport capacity.

Combining advances in the pharmacology with advances in molecular biology and protein synthesis technology have facilitated the creation of recombinant proteins, synthesized in *Escherichia coli*. These techniques have enabled investigators to modify the protein structure of the neurotoxin to create "designer" toxins with altered neuronal specificity, and may, in the future, lead to the development of neurotoxins targeted to very specific neuronal subtypes, or with altered pharmacologic properties.[64,65,66]

The development of alternative delivery systems for BoNTs has also been proposed, and clinical trials evaluating the efficacy of a topically applied neurotoxin formulation in crow's feet lines and hyperhidrosis are in development.[67,68]

1.10 Key Points/Pearls

- Botulinum neurotoxin (BoNT) is the most potent inhibitor of the release of neurotransmitters such as acetylcholine, but also inflammatory mediators such as calcitonin gene-related peptide, substance P, and glutamate.
- As a therapeutic, BoNT can be used to manage hyperfunctional muscular disorders such as dystonia, tremor, myoclonus, cosmetic facial lines, and others.
- BoNT can be used to treat pain disorders such as migraine headaches, trigeminal neuralgia, temporomandibular disorders, tension headaches, and others.
- BoNT can be used to treat autonomic disorders such as Frey syndrome, sialorrhea, sialoceles, facial hyperhidrosis, and others.

References

[1] Zornetta I, Azarnia Tehran D, Arrigoni G, et al. The first non Clostridial botulinum-like toxin cleaves VAMP within the juxtamembrane domain. Sci Rep.; 6(6):30257

[2] Peck MW, Smith TJ, Anniballi F, et al. Historical perspectives and guidelines for botulinum neurotoxin subtype nomenclature. Toxins (Basel).; 9(1):E38

[3] Masuyer G, Chaddock JA, Foster KA, Acharya KR. Engineered botulinum neurotoxins as new therapeutics. Annu Rev Pharmacol Toxicol.; 54:27–51

[4] Yao G, Lam KH, Perry K, Weisemann J, Rummel A, Jin R. Crystal structure of the receptor-binding domain of botulinum neurotoxin type HA, also known as Type FA or H. Toxins (Basel).; 9(3):1–13

[5] Popoff MR, Marvaud CC. Structural and genomic features of clostridial neurotoxins. In: Alouf J, Ladant D, Popoff M, ed. The Comprehensive Sourcebook of Bacterial Protein Toxins. 2nd ed. London: Elsevier; 1999:174–201

[6] Whitemarsh RC, Tepp WH, Bradshaw M, et al. Characterization of botulinum neurotoxin A subtypes 1 through 5 by investigation of activities in mice, in neuronal cell cultures, and in vitro. Infect Immun.; 81(10):3894–3902

[7] Pier CL, Chen C, Tepp WH, et al. Botulinum neurotoxin subtype A2 enters neuronal cells faster than subtype A1. FEBS Lett.; 585(1):199–206

[8] Torii Y, Akaike N, Harakawa T, et al. Type A1 but not type A2 botulinum toxin decreases the grip strength of the contralateral foreleg through axonal transport from the toxin-treated foreleg of rats. J Pharmacol Sci.; 117(4):275–285

[9] Torii Y, Kiyota N, Sugimoto N, et al. Comparison of effects of botulinum toxin subtype A1 and A2 using twitch tension assay and rat grip strength test. Toxicon.; 57(1):93–99

[10] Sakaguchi G. Clostridium botulinum toxins. Pharmacol Ther.; 19(2):165–194

[11] Ohishi I, Sugii S, Sakaguchi G. Oral toxicities of Clostridium botulinum toxins in response to molecular size. Infect Immun.; 16(1):107–109

[12] Kukreja RV, Singh BR. Comparative role of neurotoxin-associated proteins in the structural stability and endopeptidase activity of botulinum neurotoxin complex types A and E. Biochemistry.; 46(49):14316–14324

[13] Chen F, Kuziemko GM, Stevens RC. Biophysical characterization of the stability of the 150-kilodalton botulinum toxin, the nontoxic component, and the 900-kilodalton botulinum toxin complex species. Infect Immun.; 66(6):2420–2425

[14] DasGupta BR. Botulinum neurotoxin: studies on the structure and structure-biological activity relation. Toxicon.; 17: 41–101

[15] Smith TJ, Lou J, Geren IN, et al. Sequence variation within botulinum neurotoxin serotypes impacts antibody binding and neutralization. Infect Immun.; 73(9):5450–5457

[16] Wagman J. Isolation and sedimentation study of low molecular weight forms of type A botulins toxin. Arch Biochem Biophys.; 50(1):104–112

[17] Wagman J, Bateman JB. The behavior of the bolulinus toxins in the ultracentrifuge. Arch Biochem Biophys.; 31(3):424–430

[18] Dong M, Liu H, Tepp WH, Johnson EA, Janz R, Chapman ER. Glycosylated SV2A and SV2B mediate the entry of botulinum neurotoxin E into neurons. Mol Biol Cell.; 19(12):5226–5237

[19] Dong M, Yeh F, Tepp WH, et al. SV2 is the protein receptor for botulinum neurotoxin A. Science.; 312(5773):592–596

[20] Rummel A, Häfner K, Mahrhold S, et al. Botulinum neurotoxins C, E and F bind gangliosides via a conserved binding site prior to stimulation-dependent uptake with botulinum neurotoxin F utilising the three isoforms of SV2 as second receptor. J Neurochem.; 110(6):1942–1954

[21] Fu Z, Chen C, Barbieri JT, Kim JJ, Baldwin MR. Glycosylated SV2 and gangliosides as dual receptors for botulinum neurotoxin serotype F. Biochemistry.; 48(24):5631–5641

[22] Simpson LL. Ammonium chloride and methylamine hydrochloride antagonize clostridial neurotoxins. J Pharmacol Exp Ther.; 225(3):546–552

[23] Koriazova LK, Montal M. Translocation of botulinum neurotoxin light chain protease through the heavy chain channel. Nat Struct Biol.; 10(1):13–18

[24] Fischer A, Montal M. Crucial role of the disulfide bridge between botulinum neurotoxin light and heavy chains in protease translocation across membranes. J Biol Chem.; 282 (40):29604–29611

[25] Schiavo G, Rossetto O, Santucci A, DasGupta BR, Montecucco C. Botulinum neurotoxins are zinc proteins. J Biol Chem.; 267 (33):23479–23483

[26] Fernández-Salas E, Steward LE, Ho H, et al. Plasma membrane localization signals in the light chain of botulinum neurotoxin. Proc Natl Acad Sci U S A.; 101(9):3208–3213

[27] Foran PG, Mohammed N, Lisk GO, et al. Evaluation of the therapeutic usefulness of botulinum neurotoxin B, C1, E, and F compared with the long lasting type A. Basis for distinct durations of inhibition of exocytosis in central neurons. J Biol Chem.; 278(2):1363–1371

[28] Eleopra R, Tugnoli V, Quatrale R, Rossetto O, Montecucco C. Different types of botulinum toxin in humans. Mov Disord.; 19 Suppl 8:S53–S59

[29] de Paiva A, Meunier FA, Molgó J, Aoki KR, Dolly JO. Functional repair of motor endplates after botulinum neurotoxin type A poisoning: biphasic switch of synaptic activity between nerve sprouts and their parent terminals. Proc Natl Acad Sci U S A.; 96(6):3200–3205

[30] Meunier FA, Schiavo G, Molgó J. Botulinum neurotoxins: from paralysis to recovery of functional neuromuscular transmission. J Physiol Paris.; 96(1–2):105–113

[31] Rogozhin AA, Pang KK, Bukharaeva E, Young C, Slater CR. Recovery of mouse neuromuscular junctions from single and repeated injections of botulinum neurotoxin A. J Physiol.; 586(13):3163–3182

[32] Filippi GM, Errico P, Santarelli R, Bagolini B, Manni E. Botulinum A toxin effects on rat jaw muscle spindles. Acta Otolaryngol.; 113(3):400–404

[33] Rosales RL, Arimura K, Takenaga S, Osame M. Extrafusal and intrafusal muscle effects in experimental botulinum toxin-A injection. Muscle Nerve.; 19(4):488–496

[34] Trompetto C, Currà A, Buccolieri A, Suppa A, Abbruzzese G, Berardelli A. Botulinum toxin changes intrafusal feedback in dystonia: a study with the tonic vibration reflex. Mov Disord.; 21(6):777–782

[35] Caleo M, Antonucci F, Restani L, Mazzocchio R. A reappraisal of the central effects of botulinum neurotoxin type A: by what mechanism? J Neurochem.; 109(1):15–24

[36] McComas AJ. Oro-facial muscles: internal structure, function and ageing. Gerodontology.; 15(1):3–14

[37] Goodmurphy CW, Ovalle WK. Morphological study of two human facial muscles: orbicularis oculi and corrugator supercilii. Clin Anat.; 12(1):1–11

[38] Lowe NJ, Glaser DA, Eadie N, Daggett S, Kowalski JW, Lai PY, North American Botox in Primary Axillary Hyperhidrosis Clinical Study Group. Botulinum toxin type A in the treatment of primary axillary hyperhidrosis: a 52-week multicenter double-blind, randomized, placebo-controlled study of efficacy and safety. J Am Acad Dermatol.; 56(4):604–611

[39] Lagalla G, Millevolte M, Capecci M, Provinciali L, Ceravolo MG. Botulinum toxin type A for drooling in Parkinson's disease: a double-blind, randomized, placebo-controlled study. Mov Disord.; 21(5):704–707

[40] Kim KS, Kim SS, Yoon JH, Han JW. The effect of botulinum toxin type A injection for intrinsic rhinitis. J Laryngol Otol.; 112(3):248–251

[41] Naumann M, Zellner M, Toyka KV, Reiners K. Treatment of gustatory sweating with botulinum toxin. Ann Neurol.; 42(6):973–975

[42] Naumann M, Jost WH, Toyka KV. Botulinum toxin in the treatment of neurological disorders of the autonomic nervous system. Arch Neurol.; 56(8):914–916

[43] Dmochowski R, Chapple C, Nitti VW, et al. Efficacy and safety of onabotulinumtoxinA for idiopathic overactive bladder: a double-blind, placebo controlled, randomized, dose ranging trial. J Urol.; 184(6):2416–2422

[44] Haferkamp A, Schurch B, Reitz A, et al. Lack of ultrastructural detrusor changes following endoscopic injection of botulinum toxin type a in overactive neurogenic bladder. Eur Urol.; 46(6):784–791

[45] Greene P, Fahn S, Brin M, Moskowitz C, Flaster E. Double-blind, placebo-controlled trial of botulinum toxin injections for the treatment of spasmodic torticollis. Neurology.; 40: 1213–1218

[46] Song PC, Schwartz J, Blitzer A. The emerging role of botulinum toxin in the treatment of temporomandibular disorders. Oral Dis.; 13(3):253–260

[47] Ranoux D, Attal N, Morain F, Bouhassira D. Botulinum toxin type A induces direct analgesic effects in chronic neuropathic pain. Ann Neurol.; 64(3):274–283

[48] Piovesan EJ, Teive HG, Kowacs PA, Della Coletta MV, Werneck LC, Silberstein SD. An open study of botulinum-A toxin treatment of trigeminal neuralgia. Neurology.; 65(8):1306–1308

[49] Dodick DW, Turkel CC, DeGryse RE, et al. PREEMPT Chronic Migraine Study Group. OnabotulinumtoxinA for treatment of chronic migraine: pooled results from the double-blind, randomized, placebo-controlled phases of the PREEMPT clinical program. Headache.; 50(6):921–936

[50] Gazerani P, Pedersen NS, Staahl C, Drewes AM, Arendt-Nielsen L. Subcutaneous Botulinum toxin type A reduces capsaicin-induced trigeminal pain and vasomotor reactions in human skin. Pain.; 141(1–2):60–69

[51] Carmichael NM, Dostrovsky JO, Charlton MP. Peptide-mediated transdermal delivery of botulinum neurotoxin type A reduces neurogenic inflammation in the skin. Pain.; 149(2): 316–324

[52] Richardson JD, Vasko MR. Cellular mechanisms of neurogenic inflammation. J Pharmacol Exp Ther.; 302(3):839–845

[53] Brain SD, Williams TJ, Tippins JR, Morris HR, MacIntyre I. Calcitonin gene-related peptide is a potent vasodilator. Nature.; 313(5997):54–56

[54] McMahon SB, Bennett DLH, Bevan S. Inflammatory mediators and modulators of pain. 5th ed. Philadelphia, PA: Churchill Livingstone; 2005

[55] Latremoliere A, Woolf CJ. Central sensitization: a generator of pain hypersensitivity by central neural plasticity. J Pain.; 10(9):895–926

[56] Du J, Koltzenburg M, Carlton SM. Glutamate-induced excitation and sensitization of nociceptors in rat glabrous skin. Pain.; 89(2–3):187–198

[57] Purkiss J, Welch M, Doward S, Foster K. Capsaicin-stimulated release of substance P from cultured dorsal root ganglion neurons: involvement of two distinct mechanisms. Biochem Pharmacol.; 59(11):1403–1406

[58] Planells-Cases R, Garcìa-Sanz N, Morenilla-Palao C, Ferrer-Montiel A. Functional aspects and mechanisms of TRPV1 involvement in neurogenic inflammation that leads to thermal hyperalgesia. Pflugers Arch.; 451(1):151–159

[59] Morenilla-Palao C, Planells-Cases R, García-Sanz N, Ferrer-Montiel A. Regulated exocytosis contributes to protein kinase C potentiation of vanilloid receptor activity. J Biol Chem.; 279 (24):25665–25672

[60] Apostolidis A, Popat R, Yiangou Y, et al. Decreased sensory receptors P2X3 and TRPV1 in suburothelial nerve fibers following intradetrusor injections of botulinum toxin for human detrusor overactivity. J Urol.; 174(3):977–982, discussion 982–983

[61] Coelho A, Dinis P, Pinto R, et al. Distribution of the high-affinity binding site and intracellular target of botulinum toxin type A in the human bladder. Eur Urol.; 57(5):884–890

[62] Kaji R. Clinical differences between A1 and A2 botulinum toxin subtypes. Toxicon.; 107 Pt A:85–88

[63] Carruthers J, Solish N, Humphrey S, et al. Injectable daxibotulinumtoxin A for the treatment of glabellar lines: a phase 2, randomized, dose-ranging, double-blind, multicenter comparison with onabotulinumtoxin A and placebo. Dermatol Surg.; 43(11):321–1331

[64] Chaddock JA, Marks PM. Clostridial neurotoxins: structure-function led design of new therapeutics. Cell Mol Life Sci.; 63(5):540–551

[65] Wang J, Meng J, Lawrence GW, et al. Novel chimeras of botulinum neurotoxins A and E unveil contributions from the binding, translocation, and protease domains to their functional characteristics. J Biol Chem.; 283(25):16993–17002

[66] Meng J, Ovsepian SV, Wang J, et al. Activation of TRPV1 mediates calcitonin gene-related peptide release, which excites trigeminal sensory neurons and is attenuated by a retargeted botulinum toxin with anti-nociceptive potential. J Neurosci.; 29(15):4981–4992

[67] Brandt F, O'Connell C, Cazzaniga A, Waugh JM. Efficacy and safety evaluation of a novel botulinum toxin topical gel for the treatment of moderate to severe lateral canthal lines. Dermatol Surg.; 36 Suppl 4:2111–2118

[68] Glogau RG. Topically applied botulinum toxin type A for the treatment of primary axillary hyperhidrosis: results of a randomized, blinded, vehicle-controlled study. Dermatol Surg.; 33(1 Spec No):S76–S80

2

Botulinum Neurotoxin for Blepharospasm

Amit Patel, Andrew Blitzer, and Boris L. Bentsianov

Summary

Blepharospasm, or dystonic contractions of primarily the orbicularis oris, usually exists as a focal dystonia. Both eyes can be affected, and symptoms can be severe enough to cause functional blindness. Workup and management begin with ruling out and treatment of any underlying eye disorder such as blepharitis, conjunctivitis, or corneal irritation, and with lid hygiene and lubrication. Botulinum neurotoxin is the mainstay of treatment and is well tolerated, with dry eyes and partial ptosis being the most common side effects. Treatment can be tailored to a flexible or fixed injection schedule based on patient preference.

Keywords: blepharospasm, Meige syndrome, orbicularis oculi

2.1 Introduction

Blepharospasm is a dystonia of the facial musculature that ranges in severity from an increased blink rate to disabling contractions with pain and visual dysfunction. As with other dystonias, it is understood to be a complex neurologic disorder with abnormalities in sensory input, central processing, and motor output, interacting to produce the movement disorder.[1]

The primary muscle involved in blepharospasm is the orbicularis oculi. Other protractors of the eyelids include the corrugator superciliaris and procerus muscles. Spasms are usually bilateral but may affect one side primarily. Blepharospasm most commonly presents as a focal dystonia but can be part of a syndrome called "Meige syndrome," a segmental cranial dystonia consisting of blepharospasm with oromandibular and sometimes cervical or laryngeal dystonia (see Chapter 4).[2] Blepharospasm is uncommon, with an estimated prevalence of up to 1 case per 10,000 people. There is an increased female to male prevalence. The mean age of diagnosis is in the sixth decade of life.[3] The condition usually begins with increased blink rate or spasms of the eyelids, forehead, or midfacial muscles. Patients often complain of eye irritation, pain, photophobia, or abnormal tearing, and may initially be diagnosed with various other ocular disorders. Spasms may be triggered by sensory stimulation such as wind, air pollutants, or bright light, and may be worse in stressful situations. Some patients identify sensory tricks such as touching the face, using artificial tears, or talking and singing that may temporarily abate the spasm. The condition is often progressive and results in functional blindness in a minority of those affected.[4]

Patients may avoid social settings, reading, driving, or watching television, with ensuing anxiety and depression. Maximum disability is reached at an average of 3 years after onset.

Although severity may fluctuate, spontaneous remissions are rare. Over the long term, the persistent contractions can result in weakening of the eyelid's fascial attachments, resulting in brow ptosis, dermatochalasis, and ectropion, with further visual field obstruction. The disease typically remains focal but may involve other facial muscles or, rarely, other parts of the body.

Management begins with ruling out and treatment of any underlying eye disorder such as blepharitis, conjunctivitis, or corneal irritation, and with lid hygiene and lubrication. Tinted sunglasses with ultraviolet blocking have demonstrated efficacy as well.[5] Some patients resort to "eyelid crutches" or springs on glasses to hold lid open. Systemic medications such as benzodiazepines and the antiparkinsonian agent trihexyphenidyl (Artane) have limited efficacy and significant adverse effects.[2] Surgery is reserved for patients who fail more conservative treatments. Neurectomy of facial nerve branches has generally been abandoned in favor of myectomy of the eyelid protractors.

Botulinum neurotoxin (BoNT) injection has emerged as a treatment of choice for blepharospasm, and it is approved by the United States Food and Drug Administration (FDA) for this application. Many studies ranging from large open label to small double-blind placebo-controlled have demonstrated BoNT injection to be both effective and safe, with success rates exceeding 90%.[6,7,8,9,10,11,12,13,14] Recently, the Guideline Development Subcommittee of the American Academy of Neurology reviewed current evidence and outcomes for treatment of blepharo-spasm. Given the rise in use of different forms of BoNT, including Botox (onabotulinumtoxinA), Dysport (abobotulinumtoxinA), and Xeomin (incobotulinumtoxinA), the subcommittee also reviewed studies comparing these different formulations. Randomized controlled trials comparing Botox and Dysport showed comparable benefits between the two. Observational studies comparing long-term outcome were also reviewed, and sustained benefits were noted with Botox, Dysport, and Xeomin. Overall, they concluded that BoNT is considered the first-line treatment of blepharospasm by most movement disorder specialists and all type A toxins appear to have similar efficacy and can continue to be efficacious over long periods.[15] Other studies have examined a flexible versus fixed treatment schedule with the use of BoNT. Bladen et al found that, over a period of 10 years, flexible onabotulinumtoxin provided better long-term relief for facial dystonia than a fixed regimen. Flexible interval treatment appeared to provide better patient satisfaction and longer duration of effect compared to fixed treatment with similar complication rates.[16] Similarly, a recent cross-sectional survey of patients receiving BoNT for blepharospasm indicated that flexible, individualized treatment plans may improve satisfaction and outcomes.[17]

2.2 Workup

The diagnosis of blepharospasm is clinical, though it may initially be challenging as there is overlap between early symptoms of blepharospasm and other eye disorders. A history of other neurologic symptoms, use of psychotropic medications, and family history of dystonia should be elicited. All patients benefit from an ophthalmologic examination. Further studies and imaging should be obtained to rule out a central nervous pathology when appropriate.

Apraxia of eyelid opening is an important diagnosis that may be difficult to differentiate from blepharospasm. Like blepharospasm, it also presents with abnormal eyelid closure but is primarily due to involuntary inhibition of the levator palpebrae muscle. Examination of the lower eyelid usually shows elevation in patients with blepharospasm. This diagnosis is an important consideration when BoNT treatment fails to improve blepharospasm.[1]

2.3 Anatomy

The orbicularis oculi muscle lies in a plane just deep to the subcutaneous tissue and is divided into orbital and palpebral parts. The orbital portion forms a wide circle around the orbital rims and interdigitates with other facial muscles. It is under voluntary control and is responsible for tight closure of the eyelids. The palpebral orbicularis muscle involuntarily and gently closes the eye during blinking and sleep and is further divided into a preseptal portion that overlies the orbital septum and a pretarsal portion that extends between the medial and lateral canthi anterior to the tarsus. The skin of the eyelids is the thinnest skin in the body and contains very little subcutaneous fat. Thus, the orbicularis oculi muscle may lie just 1 mm below the surface of the skin. In the brow and cheek regions, the skin becomes considerably thicker.

2.4 Technique

Injections are performed with 1-mL syringes and 30- or 32-gauge short needles. Electromyography is not necessary to guide injection due to the consistent subcutaneous location of these muscles. The dose and exact location of each injection is tailored based on the results of previous injections. To start, onabotulinumtoxinA (Botox) is diluted to a concentration of 2.5 to 5 units (U) per 0.1 mL. The orbicularis oculi is initially treated with a somewhat low starting dose of 12 to 15 U per side, although higher doses may be required. The orbital portion of the orbicularis muscle is injected at three to six sites peripherally to the orbital rim with 2.5 to 5 U of Botox in an injection volume of 0.1 mL. It is recommended to avoid injection directly over the meridian of the eye to minimize diffusion to levator palpebrae with subsequent ptosis as well as to avoid the inferomedial orbicularis muscle to prevent diffusion to the inferior oblique muscle and to avoid interference with the lacrimal drainage apparatus (▶ Fig. 2.1; ▶ Fig. 2.2). The superior palpebral portion of the muscle is injected with 1.25 U of Botox in a volume of 0.05 mL at two sites medially and laterally, again avoiding the middle of the eyelid (▶ Fig. 2.3; ▶ Fig. 2.4).

2.5 Follow-up

Mean onset of action takes place around 3 to 5 days after injection, with peak effect at around 1 to 2 weeks. The average duration of effect is approximately 3 months, although some patients experience longer lasting relief of up to 6 months. Patients should maintain a diary of symptoms and side effects to help guide future injections. Treating physicians should carefully document each injection site and dose. Inadequate reduction of spasm should prompt an increase in dose. Injecting the pretarsal portion of the orbicularis oculi muscle with a low dose (e.g., 1.25 U of Botox) can be considered, although this may produce unwanted effects. If associated muscles such as the corrugator superciliaris and procerus muscles are involved, they may benefit from injection as well. Adverse effects (see below) indicate the need for lower doses or avoiding certain injection sites.

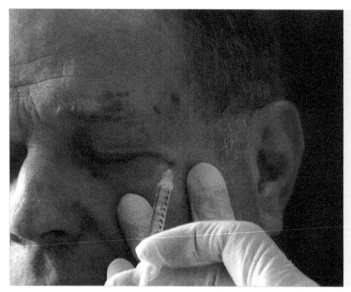

Fig. 2.1 Injection of the lateral orbital portion of the orbicularis oculi.

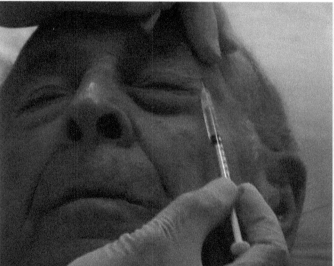

Fig. 2.2 Injection of the upper orbital portion of the orbicularis oculi.

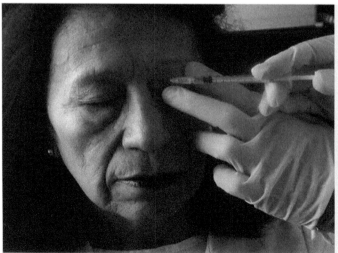

Fig. 2.3 Injection of the medial palpebral portion of the orbicularis oculi.

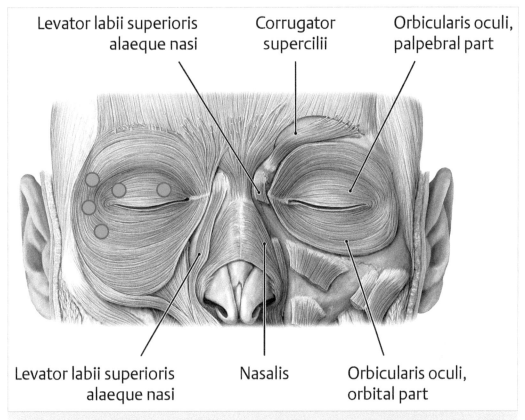

Levator labii superioris alaeque nasi   Corrugator supercilii   Orbicularis oculi, palpebral part

Levator labii superioris alaeque nasi   Nasalis   Orbicularis oculi, orbital part

Fig. 2.4 Anatomy of the orbicularis muscle, with botulinum neurotoxin injection points. (From Gilroy AM et al. Atlas of Anatomy. 1st Ed. New York: Thieme Medical Publishers; 2008. Based on: Schuenke M, Schulte E, Schumacher U. THIEME Atlas of Anatomy: Head and Neuroanatomy. Illustrations by Voll M and Wesker K. 1st Ed. New York: Thieme Medical Publishers; 2008.)

2.6 Complications and Pitfalls

Discomfort and bruising may be decreased by using smaller injection volumes and minimizing the number of injection sites. Side effects related to BoNT are more common during the early dose-optimizing period. Dry eyes and partial ptosis due to weakening of the levator palpebrae muscle are the most common side effects. Lagophthalmos may occur, and patients should be instructed to protect their eyes to prevent corneal exposure. Diplopia is rare, occurring in less than 1% of cases.[18] All of these adverse effects are generally self-limited. Proper education and informed consent are important so that patients know what to expect.

2.7 Conclusion

Blepharospasm is a debilitating neurologic disorder that can result in functional blindness. BoNT injection has emerged as a first-line treatment of choice. Knowledge of periorbital anatomy, careful attention to technique, and proper patient education are critical to obtaining good results.

2.8 Key Points/Pearls

- Blepharospasm is a dystonia of the facial musculature that ranges in severity from an increased blink rate to disabling contractions with pain and visual dysfunction.

- Workup should include a careful history and physical exam of the eye, to rule out issues such as blepharitis or eyelid apraxia.
- Treatment with BoNT involves injecting the orbicularis oculi muscle to avoid injection directly over the meridian of the eye to minimize diffusion to levator palpebrae which can cause ptosis.
- Injection over the inferomedial orbicularis muscle should be avoided to prevent diffusion to the inferior oblique muscle which can cause interference with lacrimal drainage.
- Side effects related to BoNT are more common during the early dose-optimizing period. Dry eyes and partial ptosis due to weakening of the levator palpebrae muscle are the most common side effects.

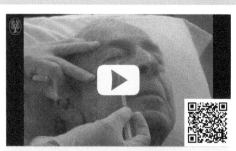

Video 2.1 Blepharospasm. An analysis of the areas of hyperfunctional muscle contraction of the orbicularis oculi is done. In general, six places are injected including two in the upper eyelid. These are placed very lateral and medial so as not to allow for migration of the toxin to the central area and the levator muscle. Weakening this muscle will produce ptosis. Additional points are injected laterally along the orbital rim. If there is a supraorbital component, then additional toxin may be given medially or laterally above the brow. [1:30]

References

[1] Hallett M, Evinger C, Jankovic J, Stacy M, BEBRF International Workshop. Update on blepharospasm: report from the BEBRF International Workshop. Neurology.; 71(16):1275–1282

[2] Jankovic J, Ford J. Blepharospasm and orofacial-cervical dystonia: clinical and pharmacological findings in 100 patients. Ann Neurol.; 13(4):402–411

[3] Defazio G, Livrea P. Epidemiology of primary blepharospasm. Mov Disord.; 17(1):7–12

[4] Jankovic J, Orman J. Botulinum A toxin for cranial-cervical dystonia: a double-blind, placebo-controlled study. Neurology.; 37(4):616–623

[5] Blackburn MK, Lamb RD, Digre KB, et al. FL-41 tint improves blink frequency, light sensitivity, and functional limitations in patients with benign essential blepharospasm. Ophthalmology.; 116(5):997–1001

[6] Truong D, Comella C, Fernandez HH, Ondo WG, Dysport Benign Essential Blepharospasm Study Group. Efficacy and safety of purified botulinum toxin type A (Dysport) for the treatment of benign essential blepharospasm: a randomized, placebo-controlled, phase II trial. Parkinsonism Relat Disord.; 14(5):407–414

[7] Silveira-Moriyama L, Gonçalves LR, Chien HF, Barbosa ER. Botulinum toxin a in the treatment of blepharospasm: a 10-year experience. Arq Neuropsiquiatr.; 63 2A:221–224

[8] Costa J, Espírito-Santo C, Borges A, et al. Botulinum toxin type A therapy for blepharospasm. Cochrane Database Syst Rev.; 1(1):CD004900

[9] Calace P, Cortese G, Piscopo R, et al. Treatment of blepharospasm with botulinum neurotoxin type A: long-term results. Eur J Ophthalmol.; 13(4):331–336

[10] Jankovic J, Schwartz K, Donovan DT. Botulinum toxin treatment of cranial-cervical dystonia, spasmodic dysphonia, other focal dystonias and hemifacial spasm. J Neurol Neurosurg Psychiatry.; 53(8):633–639

[11] Simpson DM, Blitzer A, Brashear A, et al. Therapeutics and Technology Assessment Subcommittee of the, American Academy of Neurology. Assessment: Botulinum neurotoxin for the treatment of movement disorders (an evidence-based review): report of the Therapeutics and Technology Assessment Subcommittee of the American Academy of Neurology. Neurology.; 70(19):1699–1706

[12] Jost WH, Kohl A. Botulinum toxin: evidence-based medicine criteria in blepharospasm and hemifacial spasm. J Neurol.; 248 Suppl 1:21–24

[13] Cillino S, Raimondi G, Guépratte N, et al. Long-term efficacy of botulinum toxin A for treatment of blepharospasm, hemifacial spasm, and spastic entropion: a multicentre study using two drug-dose escalation indexes. Eye (Lond).; 24(4):600–607

[14] Bentivoglio AR, Fasano A, Ialongo T, Soleti F, Lo Fermo S, Albanese A. Fifteen-year experience in treating blepharospasm with Botox or Dysport: same toxin, two drugs. Neurotox Res.; 15(3):224–231

[15] Simpson DM, Hallett M, Ashman EJ, et al. Practice guideline update summary: Botulinum neurotoxin for the treatment of blepharospasm, cervical dystonia, adult spasticity, and headache: report of the Guideline Development Subcommittee of the American Academy of Neurology. Neurology.; 86(19):1818–1826

[16] Bladen JC, Feldman I, Favor M, Dizon M, Litwin A, Malhotra R. Long-term outcome of flexible onabotulinum toxin A treatment in facial dystonia. Eye (Lond).; 33(3):349–352

[17] Fezza J, Burns J, Woodward J, Truong D, Hedges T, Verma A. A cross-sectional structured survey of patients receiving botulinum toxin type A treatment for blepharospasm. J Neurol Sci.; 367:56–62

[18] Coté TR, Mohan AK, Polder JA, Walton MK, Braun MM. Botulinum toxin type A injections: adverse events reported to the US Food and Drug Administration in therapeutic and cosmetic cases. J Am Acad Dermatol.; 53(3):407–415

3
Botulinum Neurotoxin for Facial Dystonia

Scott M. Rickert, Amy P. Wu, and Andrew Blitzer

Summary

There are many classifications of facial dystonia, including blepharospasm, oromandibular dystonia, and cervical dystonia. Meige syndrome is a combination of blepharospasm and oromandibular dystonia. Focal dystonias can occur separate from the more common syndromes and may progress to those dystonias or a more generalized dystonia. Hemifacial spasm is not a dystonia but a segmental myoclonus. Hemifacial spasm along with craniofacial tremor, facial chorea, facial tics, and facial myokymia may be initially misdiagnosed as a dystonia. It is crucial to obtain an excellent history and physical examination to distinguish these confusing entities. Botulinum toxin is a mainstay of treatment for all facial dystonia. Oral medication is frequently used in conjunction with botulinum injections but can also be used as a single treatment modality in limited cases. Surgical intervention is rare but can be helpful in the most intractable dystonias.

Keywords: facial dystonia, blepharospasm, hemifacial spasm, botulinum toxin, oromandibular dystonia, Meige syndrome, cervical dystonia, facial chorea, facial myokymia

3.1 Introduction

Dystonias of the facial region can be classified in a variety of ways. Dystonic movement disorders can affect the upper face, midface, lower face, and/or cervical region in a variety of combinations. To add to the complexity of the presentation, individual dystonias present with a variety of age ranges, frequency, and penetrance. As there is a varied presentation of dystonias of the facial/cervical region, several common facial dystonias and similar craniofacial muscle disorders are briefly described in this chapter, and basic treatment options are reviewed. Specific disorders are covered in further depth in separate chapters later in this book.

Benign essential blepharospasm or BEB is a focal dystonia that results in an involuntary closure of the musculature around the eye. BEB may include involuntary closure solely, or twitching, and repetitive movements in conjunction with closure. This involuntary movement is typically chronic and persistent in nature, resulting in a functional blindness in which there is an intact visual pathway. BEB is rare (1 in 20,000); when it occurs it tends to do so in the fifth and sixth decades of life. Botulinum neurotoxin injection to the local musculature has proven clinically effective in many reported trials.[1,2,3] The current recommendation from the American Academy of Neurology is that botulinum neurotoxin is probably effective for BEB and should be considered for first-line treatment.[4]

Hemifacial spasm, first described by Gowers in 1884, is not a dystonia but a segmental myoclonus resulting in a recurrent, involuntary, synkinetic dystonic muscular contraction of the face. The muscles in contracture are those innervated by the facial nerve and are generally unilateral as is evident in its description. There are rare cases of bilateral involvement (less than 5% per reports). It typically occurs in the fourth and fifth decades of life with a prevalence of 1 in 10,000, and usually first presents in the orbicularis oculi. The most common cause of facial nerve interruption is believed to be an aberrant vascular loop (from the posterior inferior cerebellar artery) causing local compression.[5] Other causes of compression may include local tumor, vascular malformation, and infectious processes.[6] Hemifacial spasm can be misdiagnosed as isolated blepharospasm, orbicularis oculi myokymia, or synkinetic movements post-Bell palsy. In a recent study, 62% were primary vascular causes, 2% were hereditary causes, 19% were secondary causes (Bell palsy, facial nerve injury, demyelination, brain infarcts), and 18% were mimicking causes (psychogenic, tics, dystonias, myoclonus, and hemimasticatory spasm).[7]

Given the propensity for misdiagnosis, it is important to thoroughly evaluate all dystonias for an accurate diagnosis. Anticonvulsive medication, such as oral doses of carbamazepine or valproic acid, helps control central myoclonus. Intramuscular injection of botulinum toxin reliably reduces synchronous spasms in a safe, repeatable way.[7,8,9] Defazio et al reported a 95% response rate in the effectiveness of botulinum toxin A in relieving the symptoms of primary hemifacial spasm.[10] In the case of vascular compression, surgical intervention is recommended when a localizing cause is identified.

Oromandibular dystonia (OMD) is characterized by dystonic muscular contractions affecting the jaw, mouth, and lower face. In more severe cases, the tongue musculature may be involved. In patients with OMD, involuntary contractions may involve the muscles that open the jaw, close the jaw, and the muscles of mastication. This leads to a significant variety of presentations in OMD. Associated findings may include spasms of jaw closure with difficulty opening the mouth; jaw clenching and/or bruxism; spasms of jaw opening; and sideways deviation and/or protrusion of the jaw. Additional symptoms may also be present, such as lip tightening/pursing; retraction of the corners of the mouth; and deviation and/or protrusion of the tongue. Because these findings are varied in presentation but localized, many patients with OMD may present with jaw pain, eating difficulties, or dysarthria. In a recent retrospective study, the mean age of onset was 51 years with a 2:1 female predominance with 62% having jaw-opening OMD, 20% with jaw closing, and 18% with mixed form of OMD. Lingual dystonia was present in 27% of the OMD patients.[11]

Dystonic spasms can sometimes be provoked by certain activities such as talking, chewing, or biting. There have been reported incidences of medications predicating orofacial dystonia or tardive dystonia, such as weak serotonin reuptake inhibitor, but no exact mechanism has been found.[8,11] Particular sensory tricks may help temporarily alleviate a patient's OMD symptoms. Reports of successful sensory tricks include chewing gum, talking, placing a toothpick in the mouth, lightly touching the lips or chin, or applying steady pressure in the submental region. Dystonic spasms may extend to involve nearby areas including the muscles of the eyelids, nose, neck, or vocal cords. Although some medications have been used, their efficacy is low in OMD. Botulinum toxin is the preferred treatment for all types of OMD but is most effective in the jaw closure subtype.[2] Tongue injections are contraindicated due to the risk of aspiration and supplementary oral medications are preferred for associated lingual dystonias.

Meige syndrome is the combination of blepharospasm and OMD. Presentation can be varied. It is possible for a patient to progress from a simple blepharospasm to Meige syndrome as their disease process progresses. All patients diagnosed with Meige syndrome have the presence of some component of blepharospasm and OMD. Botulinum toxin is the treatment of choice and the treatment is tailored to their symptomatology. Oral medications can help in synergy with localized botulinum toxin injections. For those patients who have medically intractable Meige syndrome, deep brain stimulation has shown efficacy in the treatment of primary Meige syndrome. In particular, deep brain stimulation to the subthalamic nucleus has improved the dystonia movement subscores from 19.3 to 5.5 and disability score from 15.6 to 6.1.[12] With these various treatments identified, Meige syndrome has several options for effective treatment.

Cervical dystonia, also known as spasmodic torticollis, is a *focal dystonia* that affects the neck and shoulders. These dystonic movements cause postural abnormalities and discomfort and can be tonic, clonic, or tonic–clonic in nature. Similar to OMD, sensory tricks can be used to relieve some of the symptoms temporarily. Physical therapy can be help-

ful but may not be fully effective in the treatment of these dystonic movements. Treatments include anticholinergic medications, and botulinum toxin injections to the affected musculature. Use of physical therapy and botulinum toxin in combination can also provide effective treatment for cervical dystonia.[13,14]

Focal dystonias exist beyond blepharospasm, OMD, and cervical dystonia. Although the majority of dystonias affecting the lower face affect the jaw as well (OMD), one can have local focal dystonia of solely the lower face or a localized region of the lower face. These focal dystonias are typically treated with local injection of botulinum toxin to the affected area every 3 to 4 months as needed.[10] Oral medications are used if the local injections are not fully effective. If the disease continues to progress, the dystonia may spread beyond its initial site, leading to a diagnosis of OMD, Meige syndrome, or even more generalized dystonias. Treatments for progressive focal dystonias are similar to those used in OMD, Meige syndrome, or generalized dystonias.[15]

Other facial manifestations of muscle contractions exist and may mimic the symptoms of a focal dystonia. Craniofacial tremor, which occurs in association with essential tremor; Parkinson disease; and electrolyte imbalances[16] are in fact focal motor seizures. The facial manifestations are typically postictal with noted weakness of the face: most often the lower face. These are typically treated by helping to treat the underlying cause of the tremor or focal motor seizure.

Facial chorea, a non-patterned movement disorder, occurs in the context of a more systemic movement disorder. Once the most systemic movement disorder is identified, the chorea can be treated in the context of the systemic movement disorder. Facial tics, on the other hand, are repetitive, partially purposeful, succinct movements of the face. Medications, physiological changes, and encephalopathy are typical causes of tic disorders and treatment of the underlying cause improves the tic disorder. Facial myokymia also presents with repetitive, succinct movements but usually begins at the vermillion border and spreads in a wave-like pattern. Myokymia is typically idiopathic and resolves over weeks to months without any further treatment.

3.2 Workup

Dystonias and dystonic-like muscular contractions of the facial region are varied in severity, nature, and location. Therefore, discerning the individual dystonia depends on the presentation. A comprehensive history and physical exam should be able to distinguish essential blepharospasm, OMD, cervical dystonia, Meige syndrome, and more localized dystonias. Other facial manifestations of musculature contractions such as craniofacial tremor, facial tics, facial chorea, facial myokymia, or hemifacial spasm may be initially misdiagnosed as dystonias. However, their subtle presentations (facial myokymia's wave-like spread pattern, craniofacial tremor's postictal presentation, repetitive facial tics, and succinct movements) should allow them to be individually identified if the history and physical is carefully examined.

3.3 Anatomy

The facial muscular anatomy is complex, with 30 individual muscles. It is important to recognize the facial musculature affected and how it can cause facial asymmetry. Whether the dystonia or dystonic-like syndrome is unilateral (hemifacial spasm), localized to the lower face (craniofacial tremor, localized OMD), or

multiple sites (Meige syndrome), identifying the individual muscles affected allows one to properly plan treatment. When creating a treatment plan for the dystonia, postinjection symmetry is also an important consideration.

3.4 Techniques/Treatments

Treatment of facial dystonias includes oral medication, intramuscular injection of botulinum toxin, and/or surgical intervention. Botulinum neurotoxin is the typical treatment of choice, but it only affects the local area of injection. Of 94 patients with cervical dystonia ($n = 33$), BEB ($n = 32$), and hemifacial spasm ($n = 29$), botulinum toxin treatment was effective in 92% of the patients.[17] Electromyography monitoring allows for better localization of the muscles affected for best efficacy of the botulinum toxin. Injections typically last 3 to 4 months and need to be repeated as the effect of botulinum toxin fades. Botulinum toxin injections have the advantage of being simple, safe, and usually indefinitely repeatable in most cases. Several open and a few controlled studies report good to excellent improvement in 76 to 100% of the patients injected of OMD and/or blepharospasm.

Oral medication (with or without physical therapy) can be used as single treatment modality or in combination with botulinum toxin for better neurological control of dystonia. When oral medications are added to a previously botulinum toxin only regimen, the amount of botulinum toxin may need to be adjusted as the medications can be synergistic in nature. Surgical intervention is rare and is reserved only for those who fail both oral medication and botulinum toxin injections in combination. Newer techniques of surgical intervention (deep brain stimulation) have preliminarily shown to have efficacy toward intractable dystonias.

3.5 Complications and Pitfalls

Complications in botulinum toxin use can occur from local diffusion or excessive response of toxin into unintended musculature. If botulinum injection diffuses into the levator muscle in a patient with blepharospasm, then it is possible to experience weakness of the levator muscle and have subsequent ptosis. If this occurs, it is possible to help stimulate the muscle with a topical sympathomimetic drug such as Apraclonidine, 0.5 to 1.0% drops. Botulinum toxin injections into an OMD patient's pterygoids, masseters, or temporalis musculature can cause excessive jaw opening and difficulty in closure. Injections near the tongue/tongue base can cause significant dysphagia and aspiration risk. Local lower face injections into the zygomaticus and risorius may flatten the nasolabial line and may change the smile and allow for an asymmetric drooping of the angle of the mouth which will be aesthetically unpleasing. These are dose-related events and may be corrected with smaller doses or asymmetric compensating injections on future visits.

3.6 Conclusion

There are many different classifications of facial dystonia, including blepharospasm, OMD, and cervical dystonia. Meige syndrome is a combination of blepharospasm and OMD. Focal dystonias can also occur separate from the more common syndromes noted and can occasionally progress to those dystonias or a more generalized dystonia. Hemifacial spasm is in fact not a dystonia but a segmental myoclonus. Hemifacial spasm along with craniofacial tremor, facial chorea, facial tics, and facial myokymia all can be initially misdiagnosed as a dystonia. It is crucial to obtain an excellent history and physical exam to distinguish these confusing entities. Botulinum toxin is a mainstay of treatment for all facial dystonias. Oral medication is frequently used in conjunction with botulinum injections, but can also be used as a single treatment modality in rare cases. Surgical intervention is rare but can be helpful in the most intractable dystonias.

3.7 Key Points/Pearls

- There are many classifications of facial dystonia, including blepharospasm, oromandibular dystonia, cervical dystonia, Meige syndrome, and focal dystonias.
- Many facial dystonias are localized to a particular area of the facial anatomy, but some may have multiple areas of the face affected at the same time.
- Other muscle contractions may mimic symptoms of dystonia but are in fact focal tremor or motor seizures.
- Given the variety of presentation, a thorough history and physical exam are essential and frequently diagnostic.
- Botulinum neurotoxin and oral medications are the mainstay of treatment for most facial dystonias.
- Thorough understanding of facial anatomy minimizes complications of botulinum injection.
- If successful, botulinum toxin injections may need to be repeated on a 3- to 4-month basis as dictated by the patient's symptoms.
- Surgical intervention is rare, but can be helpful in the most intractable dystonias.

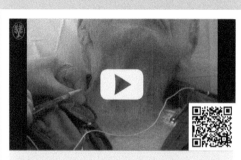

Video 3.1 Lower facial dystonia. Injecting the mentalis muscle and the depressor anguli oris will help prevent the "peau d'orange" chin and the pulling down of the corners of mouth and lower lip. Patients with lower facial dystonia may also need injections given to the upper platysma muscle to prevent excessive pull on the lower facial structures. [3:08]

References

[1] Mauriello JA. The role of botulinum toxin type A (BOTOX) in the management of blepharospasm and hemifacial spasm. In: Brin MF, Jankovic J, Hallett M, eds. Scientific and Therapeutic Aspects of Botulinum Toxin. Philadelphia, PA: Lippincott Williams & Wilkins; 2002:197–205

[2] Brin MF, Danisi F, Blitzer A. Blepharospasm, oromandibular dystonia, Meige's syndrome, and hemifacial spasm. In: Moore P, Naumann M, eds. Handbook of Botulinum Toxin Treatment, 2nd ed. Oxford, UK: Blackwell Science; 2003:119–142

[3] Defazio G, Lamberti P, Lepore V, Livrea P, Ferrari E. Facial dystonia: clinical features, prognosis and pharmacology in 31 patients. Ital J Neurol Sci.; 10(6):553–560

[4] Simpson DM, Hallett M, Ashman EJ, et al. Practice guideline update summary: Botulinum neurotoxin for the treatment of blepharospasm, cervical dystonia, adult spasticity, and headache: report of the Guideline Development Subcommittee of the American Academy of Neurology. Neurology.; 86(19):1818–1826

[5] Campos-Benitez M, Kaufmann AM. Neurovascular compression findings in hemifacial spasm. J Neurosurg.; 109(3):416–420

[6] Kraft SP, Lang AE. Cranial dystonia, blepharospasm and hemifacial spasm: treatment, including the use of botulinum toxin. CMAJ.; 139(9):837–844

[7] Mauriello JA, Jr, Leone T, Dhillon S, Pakeman B, Mostafavi R, Yepez MC. Treatment choices of 119 patients with hemifacial spasm over 11 years. Clin Neurol Neurosurg.; 98(3):213–216

[8] Yaltho TC, Jankovic J. The many faces of hemifacial spasm: differential diagnosis of unilateral facial spasms. Mov Disord.; 26(9):1582–1592

[9] Jankovic J, Schwartz K, Donovan DT. Botulinum toxin treatment of cranial-cervical dystonia, spasmodic dysphonia, other focal dystonias and hemifacial spasm. J Neurol Neurosurg Psychiatry.; 53(8):633–639

[10] Defazio G, Abbruzzese G, Girlanda P, et al. Botulinum toxin A treatment for primary hemifacial spasm: a 10-year multicenter study. Arch Neurol.; 59(3):418–420

[11] Slaim L, Cohen M, Klap P, et al. Oromandibular dystonia: demographics and clinical data from 240 patients. J Mov Disord.; 11(2):78–81

[12] Zhan S, Sun F, Pan Y, et al. Bilateral deep brain stimulation of the subthalamic nucleus in primary Meige syndrome. J Neurosurg.; 128(3):897–902

[13] Limpaphayom N, Kohan E, Huser A, Michalska-Flynn M, Stewart S, Dobbs MB. Use of combined botulinum toxin and physical therapy for treatment resistant congenital muscular torticollis. J Pediatr Orthop.; 39(5):e343–e348

[14] Borodic GE. Hemifacial spasm: evaluation and management, with emphasis on botulinum toxin therapy. In: Jankovic J, Hallett M, eds. Therapy with Botulinum Toxin. New York: Marcel Dekker; 1994:331–353

[15] Brin MF, Fahn S, Moskowitz C, et al. Localized injections of botulinum toxin for the treatment of focal dystonia and hemifacial spasm. Mov Disord.; 2(4):237–254

[16] Milton JC, Abdulla A. Prolonged oro-facial dystonia in a 58 year old female following therapy with bupropion and St John's Wort. Br J Clin Pharmacol.; 64(5):717–718

[17] Hahn K, Niklai E, Garzuly F, Szupera Z. [Botulinum toxin therapy for focal dystonia]. Orv Hetil.; 150(29):1381–1384

4
Botulinum Neurotoxin for Meige Syndrome

Niv Mor and Andrew Blitzer

Summary

Meige syndrome is a focal dystonia characterized by oromandibular dystonia with blepharospasm. Spasms are usually bilateral, symmetric, and nonrhythmic. Meige syndrome is a neurologic disorder of the basal ganglia. Although electromyography can be helpful, diagnosis is mostly based on history and physical examination. The singular use of systemic medications has often been insufficient in treating Meige syndrome. Targeted botulinum neurotoxin (BoNT) injection to the affected muscles has been most effective. The positive effects of BoNT occur over a 12-week period, and most potential side effects are mild and self-limiting. Deep brain stimulation has shown promise in suppressing dystonic brain signals and is usually reserved for cases where BoNT injections have been ineffective.

Keywords: Meige syndrome, oromandibular dystonia, blepharospasm, electromyography, botulinum neurotoxin, dystonia

4.1 Introduction

Meige syndrome is a rare focal dystonia characterized by oromandibular dystonia (OMD) and blepharospasm. The disorder was first described in 1910 by the French neurologist Henry Meige. Most cases occur in the sixth decade of life and are twice as common in women than in men. Although symptoms are typically first seen between 30 and 70 years of age, cases have been reported in younger individuals. Muscle spasms usually progress gradually and increase in intensity to incorporate more muscle groups over a period of 1 to 4 years.[1]

4.2 Symptoms

The orofacial spasms associated with Meige syndrome are usually bilateral, symmetric, and nonrhythmic lasting from seconds to minutes. Blepharospasm results in involuntary blinking sometimes causing eye irritation or dry eyes.[2] Symptoms often occur in response to bright lights, emotional stress, wind, air pollution, or other stimuli. Blepharospasm can start unilaterally but often progresses to include both eyes. Severe cases may result in involuntary eye closure. OMD is often seen as involuntary contractions of the jaw. Patients often have difficulty either opening or closing their mouth and can present with jaw clenching, teeth grinding, or repeated lip pursing. In some cases, the tongue and throat is affected resulting in tongue protrusion, dysphagia, or dyspnea.[3]

4.3 Pathophysiology

The exact symptomatology and severity of Meige syndrome varies for each individual. Historically, the disorder was considered psychogenic in origin. While symptoms are susceptible to psychosocial stressors, the condition is generally understood as neurologic in origin and resulting from a combination of genetic and environmental factors. Secondary Meige syndrome can occur in the context of neurodegenerative disorders, after the chronic administration of neuroleptics or in patients with focal brain lesions. Cases of secondary Meige syndrome have helped localize the disorder to the basal ganglia or the mesencephalic/diencephalic region of the central nervous system.[4] A study using functional magnetic resonance imaging (fMRI) showed reduced activation of the primary motor and ventral precortex during involuntary oromandibular movements in addition to increased activation of the somatosensory cortex. These findings likely reflect reduced cortical inhibition in motor and premotor cortex in combination with altered somatosensory activity.[5]

4.4 Workup

The diagnosis of Meige syndrome is based on a comprehensive history and physical examination focusing on the ophthalmologic, otolaryngologic, and neurologic systems. A patient's medication history may reveal the presence of other neurological disorders or highlight any risk factors for secondary Meige syndrome. A thorough family history focusing on the presence of other neurologic disorders is also important.

Next, it is essential to adequately identify the specific affected muscles. Attention should be given to orbicularis oris, depressor anguli oris, orbicularis oculi, temporalis, masseter, platysma, and pterygoid muscles (▶ Fig. 4.1).

Once the affected muscles are identified, objective confirmation using electromyography (EMG) can also be performed. Consultation with a neurologist who specializes in the treatment of movement disorders will be helpful in starting the patient on any appropriate oral medications and in identifying any additional neurologic symptoms. Consultation with an ophthalmologist will be helpful in establishing the patient's baseline vision and assessing if any ophthalmologic treatment will be required. Lastly, one may consider consultation with a dentist specializing in oral physiology to see if there has been any adverse effect on the patient's dentition or dental health.[6]

4.5 Treatment

Treatments with systemic medications have often been unsatisfactory and temporary. Nonetheless, approximately one-third of patients are treated with systemic neurologic agents. Some systemic medications include dopaminergic/anticholinergics, tetrabenazine, benzodiazepines, and baclofen. Ablative surgery has proven to be ineffective and is no longer utilized as acceptable treatment. Historically, ablative surgery was limited to controlling blepharospasm and included eyelid myectomy, blepharoplasty, and lid lifts. Patients with refractory primary generalized dystonia have shown remarkable symptom improvement with globus pallidus deep brain stimulation (DBS).[7,8] Botulinum neurotoxin (BoNT) injections directed at the affected muscles have shown great success in controlling patients' associated muscle spasms.

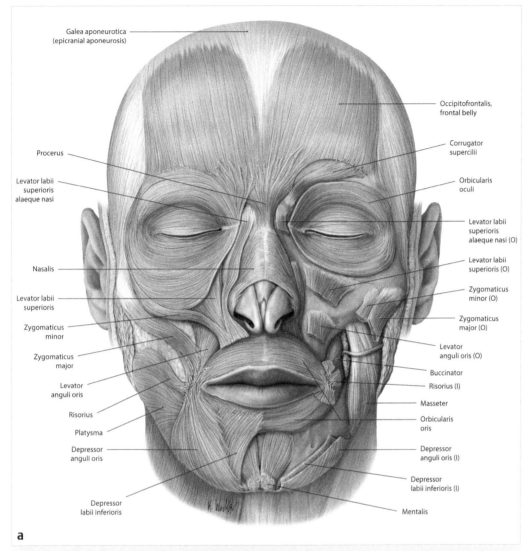

Galea aponeurotica
(epicranial aponeurosis)

Procerus

Levator labii
superioris
alaeque nasi

Nasalis

Levator labii
superioris

Zygomaticus
minor

Zygomaticus
major

Levator
anguli oris

Risorius

Platysma

Depressor
anguli oris

Depressor
labii inferioris

Occipitofrontalis,
frontal belly

Corrugator
supercilii

Orbicularis
oculi

Levator labii
superioris
alaeque nasi (O)

Levator labii
superioris (O)

Zygomaticus
minor (O)

Zygomaticus
major (O)

Levator
anguli oris (O)

Buccinator

Risorius (I)

Masseter

Orbicularis
oris

Depressor
anguli oris (I)

Depressor
labii inferioris (I)

Mentalis

a

Fig. 4.1 (a) Front view of muscle anatomy with attention to orbicularis oculi, orbicularis oris, depressor anguli oris, temporalis, masseter, and platysma muscles. (From Gilroy AM et al. Atlas of Anatomy. 1st Ed. New York: Thieme Medical Publishers; 2008. Based on: Schuenke M, Schulte E, Schumacher U. THIEME Atlas of Anatomy: Head and Neuroanatomy. Illustrations by Voll M and Wesker K. 1st Ed. New York: Thieme Medical Publishers; 2008.) (*Continued*)

4.6 Deep Brain Stimulation

Although the exact mechanism of action for DBS is not fully understood, DBS has been shown to decrease patients' symptoms by suppressing the excessive brain signals seen in dystonia.[9] DBS is not appropriate for all patients and not all patients will have the same results. Generally, patients experience 50 to 60% reduction of

symptoms following DBS. Some patients have reported 80 to 90% reduction of symptoms. Results have been sustained with some experiencing improvement up to 20 years following surgery.[9] Younger patients who arepositive for the DYT1 gene mutation who are treated earlier for the progression of the disorder have had better results than those with nongenetic acquired dystonia.[9,10,11] Results with DBS

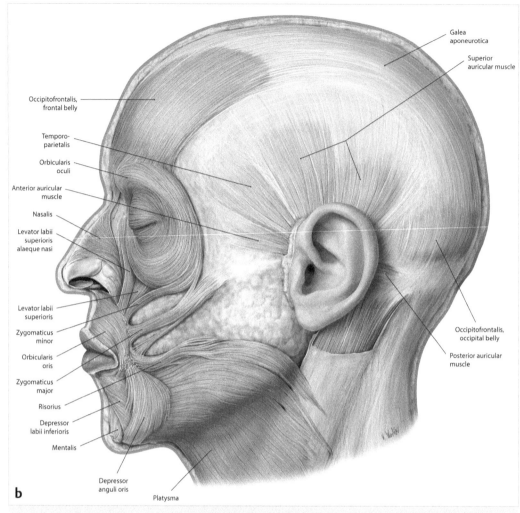

Fig. 4.1 (b) Side view of muscle anatomy with attention to orbicularis oculi, orbicularis oris, depressor anguli oris, temporalis, masseter, and platysma muscles. (From Gilroy AM et al. Atlas of Anatomy. 1st Ed. New York: Thieme Medical Publishers; 2008. Based on: Schuenke M, Schulte E, Schumacher U. THIEME Atlas of Anatomy: Head and Neuroanatomy. Illustrations by Voll M and Wesker K. 1st Ed. New York: Thieme Medical Publishers; 2008.)

to treat focal cranial nerve dystonia, including blepharospasm and OMD, have also been promising.[9] DBS is usually reserved for cases of severe dystonia when other treatments, such as BoNT injections, have been ineffective.

4.7 Injection Technique

Targeted BoNT injection is safe and effective at ameliorating the dystonic movements associated with Meige syndrome and can be used separately or in combi-nation with systemic medication. The most common muscles treated with BoNT are the orbicularis oculi, orbicularis oris, depressor anguli oris, temporalis, masseter, lateral pterygoid, and platysma muscles.

4.7.1 Temporalis Muscle and Masseter Muscle

Injection to the temporalis and masseter muscles is performed under the guid-ance of EMG. We perform injections using a 27-gauge EMG-guided monopolar electrode injection needle. If possible, patients are asked to clench their teeth to aid in EMG localization. A starting dose of 10 to 25 units is given to each temporalis muscle and 25 to 50 units to each masseter muscle. A dilution of 5.0 units per 0.1 mL is delivered at 0.1 mL aliquots. Injections are spaced at least 1 cm apart to account for the diffusion properties of BoNT. When administering the injection to the masseter muscle, the needle should be directed laterally to minimize diffusion of BoNT to nearby muscles of facial expression (▶ Fig. 4.2).[12,13]

4.7.2 Lateral Pterygoid Muscle

Injection to the lateral pterygoid muscle is performed under EMG guidance and can be approached intraorally or extraorally. For the intraoral approach, the needle is placed between the pterygoid plate and the coronoid process of the mandible (▶ Fig. 4.3). EMG confirmation of intramuscular injection is obtained by audible signals heard with lateral jaw movements, and injection is performed as the needle is withdrawn. In this fashion, injection is achieved along the length of the muscle.[12] For the extraoral approach, the location of condyle head is palpated as the patient moves their jaw laterally. The needle is advanced at a 45-angle posteriorly to engage the condylar head. The needle is then advanced anteriorly and deep until audible signaling is established. Similar to the interoral approach, confirmation is obtained by

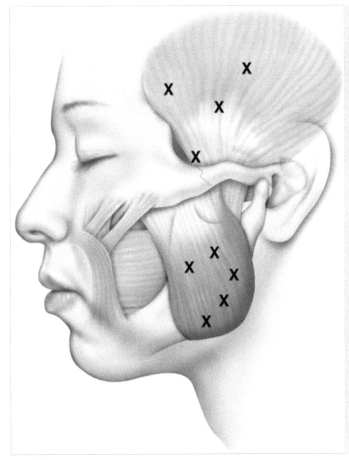

Fig. 4.2 Needle placement for injection of botulinum toxin to the temporalis and masseter muscles. (Used with permission from Bentsianov B, Francis A, Blitzer A. Botulinum toxin treatment of temporomandibular disorders, masseteric hypertrophy, and cosmetic masseter reduction. Oper Tech Otolaryng Head Neck Surg 2004;15 (2):110–113.)

lateral jaw movements prior to injecting BoNT.[14] A dilution of 2.5 units per 0.1 mL is used for the lateral pterygoid muscle with a starting does of 7.5 to 10 units per side.

4.7.3 Orbicularis Oris and Depressor Anguli Oris

Orbicularis oris and depressor anguli oris muscles are superficially located and thus EMG guidance is not necessary when injecting these muscle groups. When injecting orbicularis oris, one should avoid injecting directly over the meridian of the eye to reduce the risk of diffusion to the levator palpebrae and subsequent development of ptosis. One should also avoid injecting near the inferomedial orbicularis oculi muscle to limit diffusion to the inferior oblique muscle. The location of the depressor anguli oris can be found at a point 7 mm lateral and 7 mm inferior to the oral commissure.[15] Injection of 2 to 4 units at this location is usually sufficient (▶ Fig. 4.1; ▶ Fig. 4.4).

4.7.4 Platysma Muscle

Injection to the platysma muscle can be performed under EMG guidance. The anterior and posterior border of the platysma muscle is identified and marked by horizontal lines spanning the width of

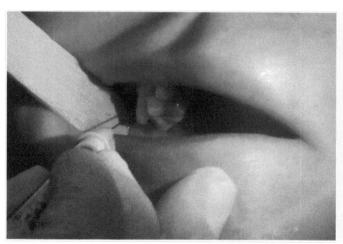

Fig. 4.3 Intraoral electromyography-guided injection of botulinum toxin to the lateral pterygoid muscle.

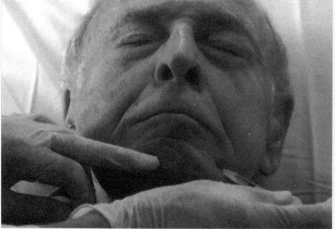

Fig. 4.4 Transcutaneous injection of botulinum toxin to the depressor anguli oris muscle.

the muscle. Parallel lines are marked 2 cm apart until the bottom of the platysma muscle is reached (▶ Fig. 4.5).

An EMG-guided injection needle is then placed at the anterior edge until muscle activity is heard. The needle is then directed parallel to the skin and posteriorly, along the delineated horizontal line at the level of the muscle fibers.[15] Injection is then given through the muscle as the needle is withdrawn (▶ Fig. 4.6).

Typically three to four injections per side are administered with each pass delivering 2.5 to 5.0 units of BoNT. An alternative technique to injecting the platysma muscle is along the vertical bands. The patient activates the platysma muscle and each vertical band is injected with the same aforementioned dose (▶ Fig. 4.7).

4.8 Follow-up

The onset of action of BoNT occurs 3 to 5 days after the initial injection, and the duration of efficacy usually lasts 12 weeks. Some variability with respect to dosing frequency has been noted with some patients experiencing longer lasting relief of up to 6 months. Patients usually return for reevaluation approximately 3 to 4 weeks after the initial injection for an interval

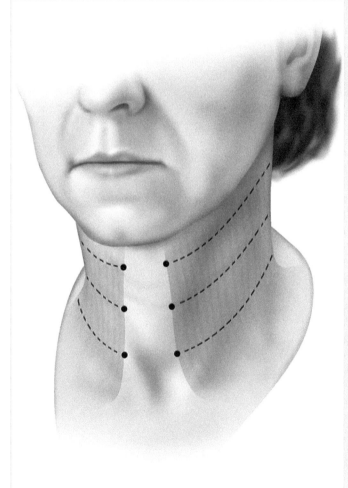

Fig. 4.5 Platysma muscles marked by horizontal lines spanning the width of the muscle. (Used with permission from Wynn R, Bentsianov B, Blitzer A. Botulinum toxin injection for the lower face and neck. Oper Tech Otolaryng Head Neck Surg 2004;12:139–142.)

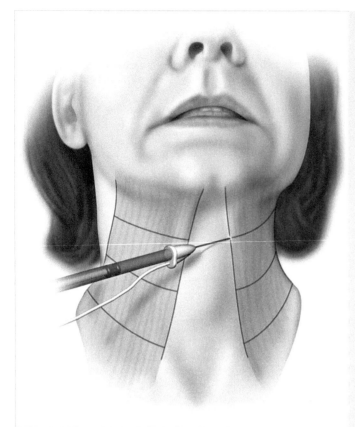

Fig. 4.6 Transcutaneous injection of botulinum toxin along the delineated horizontal lines. (Used with permission from Wynn R, Bentsianov B, Blitzer A. Botulinum toxin injection for the lower face and neck. Oper Tech Otolaryng Head Neck Surg 2004;12:139–142.)

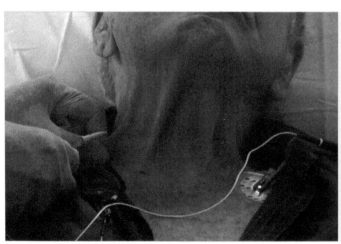

Fig. 4.7 Transcutaneous injection of botulinum toxin to vertical platysma muscle bands.

checkup. Physicians should document each injection site and dose and the patient should maintain a diary of symptoms and side effects. Some patients may require a booster injection at that time. Once the initial dose is optimized, follow-up injections occur every 12 weeks. It is important to note that an individual patient's response to toxin may change over time, and thus we advocate for patient-directed dosing with dose adjustment based on the patient's response to the previous injection cycle.[12]

4.9 Complications

Side effects related to BoNT injection are more common during the initial dose-optimization period and most are self-limiting. Discomfort and bruising at the injection site may be treated with subsequent smaller dose volumes and reduction in the number of injection sites. Dry eyes and ptosis may result from weakness of the levator palpebrae muscle following injection of orbicularis oculi. Patients should protect their eyes to prevent corneal abrasion should lagophthalmos occur. Diplopia is a rare side effect but can occur in less than 1% of patients. Difficulty chewing is the most common adverse side effect from injection to temporalis, masseter, and pterygoid muscles. Muscle atrophy may result in poor cosmesis. Paralysis or paresis to the muscles of facial expression may occur if the masseter muscle is injected too close to the zygomaticus major.[16,17,18,19] Dry mouth may occur if BoNT is injected into the parotid gland. Flulike symptoms are rarely seen and are usually self-limiting and brief.

4.10 Conclusion

Meige syndrome is a rare adult-onset focal dystonia characterized by **OMD** and blepharospasm. EMG-guided **BoNT** injections targeted at the specific affected muscles is a safe and effective treatment to ameliorate the dystonic movements associated with Meige syn-

drome. DBS is a safe and effective treatment option in medically refractory dystonia and is usually reserved for cases where BoNT injections have been ineffective.

4.11 Key Points/Pearls

- Meige syndrome is a focal oromandibular dystonia with blepharospasm.
- Primary Meige syndrome is a neurologic disorder of the basal ganglion.
- Secondary Meige syndrome can result from neurodegenerative disorders, following long-term use of neuroleptics or in patients with brain lesions.
- The diagnosis of Meige syndrome is based on a comprehensive history and physical examination.
- Electromyography (EMG) can be helpful in providing objective confirmation of the diagnosis.
- Systemic medications have often been unsatisfactory in treating Meige syndrome.
- Targeted botulinum neurotoxin (BoNT) injections to the affected muscles have been most effective.
- Patients often require planned serial BoNT injections every 12 weeks.
- Targeted treatment to the affected muscle is often aided with EMG-guided BoNT injections.
- The most commonly treated muscles are the orbicularis oculi, orbicularis oris, depressor anguli oris, temporalis, masseter, lateral pterygoid, and platysma muscles.
- Most potential side effects are mild and self-limiting.
- Deep brain stimulation has shown promise in refractory cases.

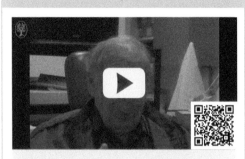

Video 4.1 Meige syndrome (multicranial dystonia). Notice this patient's excessive blinking, pulling of lower facial muscles, platysma, and anterior neck. He also has intermittent dysarthria. [0:26]

References

[1] DeLong MR. Oromandibular dystonia and Meige syndrome. NORD Guide to Rare Disorders.. Philadelphia, PA: Lippincott Williams & Wilkins; 2003:615–616

[2] Tsubota K, Fujihara T, Kaido M, Mori A, Mimura M, Kato M. Dry eye and Meige's syndrome. Br J Ophthalmol.; 81(6): 439–442

[3] Tolosa ES. Clinical features of Meige's disease (idiopathic orofacial dystonia): a report of 17 cases. Arch Neurol.; 38(3): 147–151

[4] Tolosa E, Martí MJ. Blepharospasm-oromandibular dystonia syndrome (Meige's syndrome): clinical aspects. Adv Neurol.; 49:73–84

[5] Dresel C, Haslinger B, Castrop F, Wohlschlaeger AM, Ceballos-Baumann AO. Silent event-related fMRI reveals deficient motor and enhanced somatosensory activation in orofacial dystonia. Brain.; 129(Pt 1):36–46

[6] Møller E, Werdelin LM, Bakke M, Dalager T, Prytz S, Regeur L. Treatment of perioral dystonia with botulinum toxin in 4 cases of Meige's syndrome. Oral Surg Oral Med Oral Pathol Oral Radiol Endod.; 96(5):544–549

[7] Markaki E, Kefalopoulou Z, Georgiopoulos M, Paschali A, Constantoyannis C. Meige's syndrome: A cranial dystonia treated with bilateral pallidal deep brain stimulation. Clin Neurol Neurosurg.; 112(4):344–346

[8] Houser M, Waltz T. Meige syndrome and pallidal deep brain stimulation. Mov Disord.; 20(9):1203–1205

[9] Meoni S, Fraix V, Castrioto A, et al. Pallidal deep brain stimulation for dystonia: a long term study. J Neurol Neurosurg Psychiatry.; 88(11):960–967

[10] Volkmann J, Wolters A, Kupsch A, et al. DBS study group for dystonia. Pallidal deep brain stimulation in patients with primary generalised or segmental dystonia: 5-year follow-up of a randomised trial. Lancet Neurol.; 11(12):1029–1038

[11] Andrews C, Aviles-Olmos I, Hariz M, Foltynie T. Which patients with dystonia benefit from deep brain stimulation? A metaregression of individual patient outcomes. J Neurol Neurosurg Psychiatry.; 81(12):1383–1389

[12] Mor N, Tang C, Blitzer A. Temporomandibular myofacial pain treated with botulinum toxin injection. Toxins (Basel).; 7(8): 2791–2800

[13] Bentsianov B, Francis A, Blitzer A. Botulinum toxin treatment of temporomandibular disorders, masseteric hypertrophy, and cosmetic masseter reduction. Oper Tech Otolaryngol–Head Neck Surg.; 15(2):110–113

[14] Sunil Dutt C, Ramnani P, Thakur D, Pandit M. Botulinum toxin in the treatment of muscle specific oro-facial pain: a literature review. J Maxillofac Oral Surg.; 14(2):171–175

[15] Wynn R, Bentsianov B, Blitzer A. Botulinum toxin injection for the lower face and neck. Oper Tech Otolaryngol–Head Neck Surg.; 12:139–142

[16] Pomprasit M, Chintrakarn C. Treatment of Frey's syndrome with botulinum toxin. J Med Assoc Thai.; 90(11):2397–2402

[17] Shilpa PS, Kaul R, Sultana N, Bhat S. Botulinum toxin: the Midas touch. J Nat Sci Biol Med.; 5(1):8–14

[18] D'Elia JB, Blitzer A. Temporomandibular disorders, masseteric hypertrophy, and cosmetic masseter reduction. In: Blitzer A, Benson BE, Guss J, eds. Botulinum Neurotoxin for Head and Neck Disorders. 1st ed. New York, NY: Thieme; 2012;141–151

[19] Nixdorf DR, Heo G, Major PW. Randomized controlled trial of botulinum toxin A for chronic myogenous orofacial pain. Pain.; 99(3):465–473

5
Botulinum Neurotoxin for Oromandibular Dystonia

Daniel Novakovic and Ajay E. Chitkara

Summary

Oromandibular dystonia (OMD) can affect various muscle groups in the mouth, face, and head. This disorder can alter speech, mastication, and swallowing. OMD can be treated with directed injections of botulinum toxin (BoNT) to specific, involved muscles. Symptom response to the BoNT injections is variable and can be related to the affected muscles.

Keywords: oromandibular dystonia, Meige syndrome, jaw dystonia, tongue dystonia, masseter dystonia, botulinum toxin

5.1 Introduction

Oromandibular dystonia or OMD is a neurologic disorder affecting both males and females with onset primarily in the fifth and sixth decades of life. It is characterized by repetitive, involuntary, patterned contractions or spasms of the masticatory, lingual, and perioral musculature. Typically, the dystonic movements are action induced and can impair speech, mastication, and swallowing, and cause significant social embarrassment. OMD is a subset of cranial-cervical dystonias, and when the symptoms of OMD are coupled with blepharospasm, the condition is known as Meige syndrome. Like other focal dystonias, it is usually a primary condition related to an underlying disorder at the levels of the basal ganglia and cerebellum. However, it may also occur secondary to other causes such as drug exposure (especially neuroleptics), Wilson disease, and peripheral injury such as dental procedures.[1,2,3,4]

Oromandibular dystonia may be classified as jaw opening, jaw closing, jaw deviation, and tongue protrusion subtypes, with most cases representing a combination of these subtypes. Perioral movements (depressor anguli oris [DAO], platysma) and head turning (sternocleidomastoid muscle [SCM]) may also be associated, but it is not clear whether they are compensatory to the OMD or part of a more complex multifocal dystonia such as Meige syndrome.

5.2 Workup

Patients should be evaluated for a family history of dystonia or the presence of other dystonias. A detailed drug and psychiatric history is also very important to exclude the possibility of tardive dystonia secondary to dopaminergic antagonists or neuroleptic drugs.[1] Some OMDs may be alleviated by a sensory trick,[5] or *geste antagoniste*, such as singing, chewing on a toothpick, placing an olive pit into the gingivobuccal sulcus, or scratching the chin. These sensory tricks afford temporary symptomatic relief. However, custom oral appliances may significantly benefit patients with jaw-opening OMD and can eliminate the need for botulinum toxin injections in some patients.[6,7]

Oral agents may be used as first-line treatment for OMD; these show benefit in approximately one-third of these patients.[8] Evaluation by a neurologist for consideration of such treatment is a prudent initial step. Botulinum neurotoxin (BoNT) injections can also be used to reduce or eliminate involuntary movements and are well established as a treatment since their first description by Brin et al and Blitzer et al[9,10] in 1987. Patients with jaw-closing OMD tend to respond better than patients with the other types of dystonic movements. Imaging may reveal evidence of prior head trauma or abnormality of the basal ganglia or cerebellum. Blood tests are not routinely performed prior to initiation of BoNT therapy, although low serum ceruloplasmin and certain genetic markers may be consistent with the diagnosis of dystonia.

5.3 Selection of Treatment Areas and Injection Anatomy

5.3.1 Jaw Deviation/Protrusion

Involuntary spasms of the external (lateral) pterygoid muscles are responsible for jaw-deviation and jaw-protrusion movements. Treatment of these OMD movements begins with injecting the external pterygoids. This muscle consists of two heads; the superior head originates on the greater wing of the sphenoid bone, and the inferior head originates on the lateral surface of the lateral pterygoid plate and runs posterolateral. The superior and inferior heads converge to insert into the medial aspect of the condylar process of the mandible (▶ Fig. 5.1).

Unilateral action of these muscles causes lateral jaw excursion to the contralateral side. Bilateral action of these muscles causes jaw protrusion or jaw

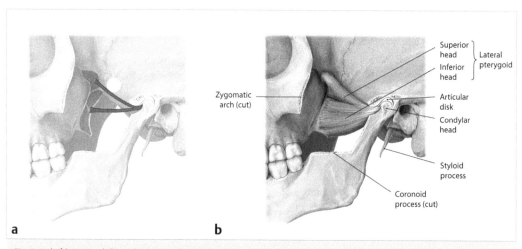

a   b

Fig. 5.1 (a,b) External (lateral) pterygoid muscle. (From Gilroy AM et al. Atlas of Anatomy. 1st Ed. New York: Thieme Medical Publishers; 2008. Based on: Schuenke M, Schulte E, Schumacher U. THIEME Atlas of Anatomy: Head and Neuroanatomy. Illustrations by Voll M and Wesker K. 1st Ed. New York: Thieme Medical Publishers; 2008.)

opening. The internal (medial) pterygoids are primarily jaw closers but can work with the external pterygoids in jaw deviation (▶ Fig. 5.2). The anterior aspect of the temporalis muscles may also be targeted to treat jaw-deviation–related dystonia.[8]

5.3.2 Jaw Closing

Involuntary actions of the masseter, temporalis, and internal or medial pterygoid muscles are responsible for jaw-closing

OMD movements (▶ Fig. 5.3). Initial treatment involves injecting the masseter and temporalis muscles first and adding treatment of the internal pterygoid for nonresponsive cases or suboptimal results.

The masseter originates from the anterior two-thirds of the zygomatic arch and the zygomatic process of the maxilla. It inserts on the inferior and lateral surface of the angle and lower ramus of the mandible (▶ Fig. 5.4). The internal (or medial) pterygoid originates from the

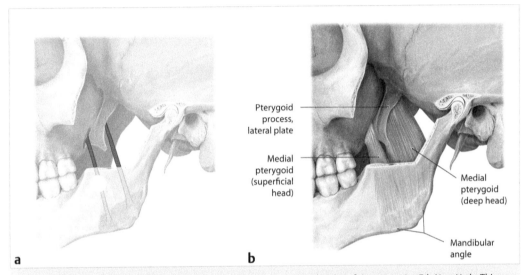

Fig. 5.2 (a,b) Internal (medial) pterygoid muscle. (From Gilroy AM et al. Atlas of Anatomy. 1st Ed. New York: Thieme Medical Publishers; 2008. Based on: Schuenke M, Schulte E, Schumacher U. THIEME Atlas of Anatomy: Head and Neuroanatomy. Illustrations by Voll M and Wesker K. 1st Ed. New York: Thieme Medical Publishers; 2008.)

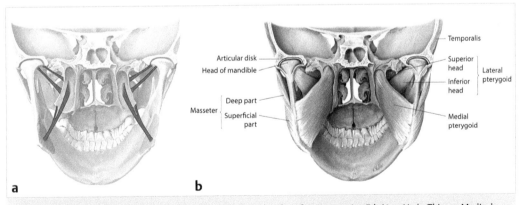

Fig. 5.3 (a,b) Muscles of mastication. (From Gilroy AM et al. Atlas of Anatomy. 1st Ed. New York: Thieme Medical Publishers; 2008. Based on: Schuenke M, Schulte E, Schumacher U. THIEME Atlas of Anatomy: Head and Neuroanatomy. Illustrations by Voll M and Wesker K. 1st Ed. New York: Thieme Medical Publishers; 2008.)

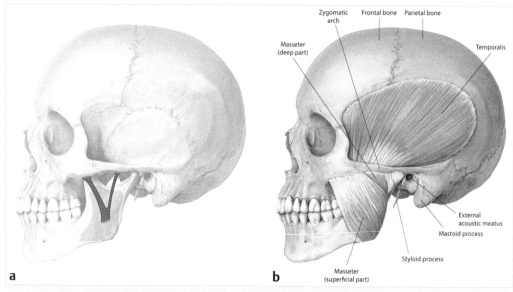

Fig. 5.4 (a,b) Masseter muscle. (From Gilroy AM et al. Atlas of Anatomy. 1st Ed. New York: Thieme Medical Publishers; 2008. Based on: Schuenke M, Schulte E, Schumacher U. THIEME Atlas of Anatomy: Head and Neuroanatomy. Illustrations by Voll M and Wesker K. 1st Ed. New York: Thieme Medical Publishers; 2008.)

medial surface of the lateral pterygoid plate, pyramidal process of palatine bone, and maxillary tuberosity. It inserts on the medial angle of the mandible, forming a U-shaped sling around the inferior mandible border with the masseter. These two muscles elevate the mandible, enabling forced closure of the mouth.

The temporalis muscle is a broad fan-shaped muscle originating from the temporal lines on the parietal bone of the skull and inserting into the coronoid process of the mandible after passing medial to the zygomatic arch. It is covered by a strong thick fascia that can be felt as resistance when administering injections. It elevates and retracts the mandible (▶ Fig. 5.5).

The jaw-closing muscles are characterized by larger masses of contractile tissue[11] compared with the jaw-opening muscles and accordingly require larger doses of BoNT. They respond better to BoNT treatment compared with the jaw-opening OMDs.[12]

5.3.3 Jaw Opening/Tongue Movements

The OMDs of jaw opening are mostly due to involuntary movements of the submental muscles (digastrics, genioglossus, geniohyoid, mylohyoid, hyoglossus) and the external pterygoids (▶ Fig. 5.6). The platysma can also function as a jaw opener, and its treatment is addressed in Chapter 9 of this book.

The digastric muscle has two bellies that insert into an intermediate tendon on the greater horn of the hyoid bone. The anterior belly originates from the digastric fossa on the anterior internal mandible, and the posterior belly originates from the mastoid process of the temporal bone. The muscles open the jaw when the temporalis and masseter are relaxed.

The genioglossus, geniohyoid, mylohyoid, and hyoglossus have lesser effects on jaw opening, but all assist in tongue movement and deglutition. Treatment of these muscles can be very challenging

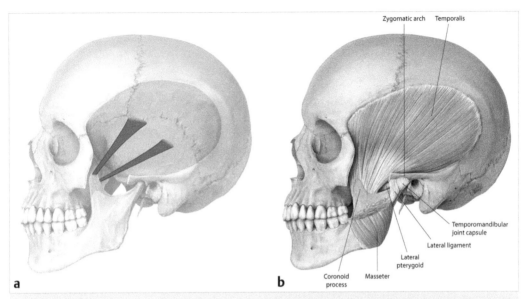

Fig. 5.5 (a,b) Temporalis muscle. (From Gilroy AM et al. Atlas of Anatomy. 1st Ed. New York: Thieme Medical Publishers; 2008. Based on: Schuenke M, Schulte E, Schumacher U. THIEME Atlas of Anatomy: Head and Neuroanatomy. Illustrations by Voll M and Wesker K. 1st Ed. New York: Thieme Medical Publishers; 2008.)

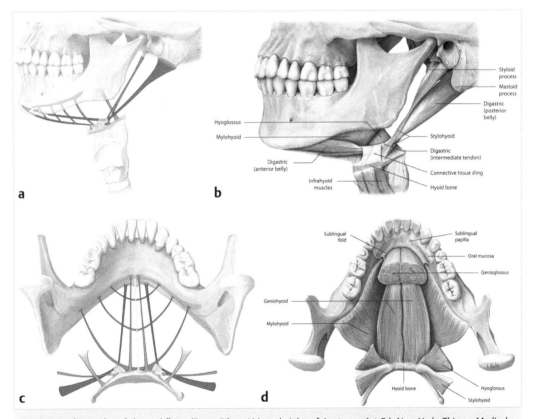

Fig. 5.6 (a–d) Muscles of the oral floor. (From Gilroy AM et al. Atlas of Anatomy. 1st Ed. New York: Thieme Medical Publishers; 2008. Based on: Schuenke M, Schulte E, Schumacher U. THIEME Atlas of Anatomy: Head and Neuroanatomy. Illustrations by Voll M and Wesker K. 1st Ed. New York: Thieme Medical Publishers; 2008.)

due to the high risk of dysphagia and dysarthria (over 10%) due to overinjection, diffusion, or inaccurate needle placement. The normal flaccid paresis from the BoNT can also cause undesirable effects on mastication and speech.

5.3.4 Tongue Movements

Tongue movements in OMD may be due primarily to extrinsic or intrinsic tongue musculature involvement or secondarily to movements of the jaw. Tongue protrusion movements are the most common and most symptomatic for the patient. When OMD results predominantly in tongue protrusion, treatment with BoNT injections into the genioglossus muscles (▶ Fig. 5.7) can improve symptoms in two-thirds of patients with an approximate 15% rate of mild dysphagia.[13] These injections should be utilized cautiously

in select cases when lingual protrusion as part of OMD persists despite treatment of jaw movements. The high risk of dysphagia and the potential for nasogastric or gastrostomy tube placement secondary to genioglossal chemodenervation[14] preclude the routine use of these injections.

5.4 Injection Technique

Patients are seated comfortably in a procedural chair. All injections are complemented with electromyographic (EMG) guidance. Ground and reference electrodes are placed over the SCM in the neck. Local anesthesia is not routinely used. Injections are performed using a hollow, 27-gauge, 37-mm-long, Teflon-coated, monopolar EMG needle placed on a 1-mL tuberculin syringe. The areas of skin overlying the muscles to be treated

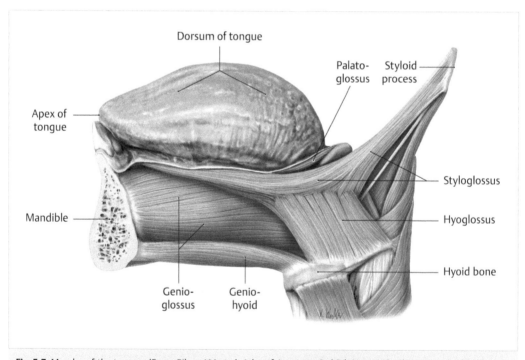

Fig. 5.7 Muscles of the tongue. (From Gilroy AM et al. Atlas of Anatomy. 3rd Ed. New York: Thieme Medical Publishers; 2016. Based on: Schuenke M, Schulte E, Schumacher U. THIEME Atlas of Anatomy: Head and Neuroanatomy. Illustrations by Voll M and Wesker K. 1st Ed. New York: Thieme Medical Publishers; 2008.)

are prepared using alcohol. To minimize the risk of contamination, the intraoral injections are administered last.

5.4.1 Masseter

A dilution of 5 units (U) per 0.1 mL of onabotulinumtoxinA is used for the masseter. The muscle belly can be palpated prior to injection by asking the patient to clench the teeth. The needle is placed through the skin into the muscle, and the position is confirmed by listening for brisk EMG activity while the patient clenches his or her teeth (▶ Fig. 5.8). The procedure is repeated on the contralateral side. A nearly perpendicular injection angle is used to deliver 0.1-mL aliquots at three or four sites in the muscle. Prior to withdrawing the needle from the skin, injections are dispersed within the muscle by changing the depth and angle of the needle. The injections are spaced approximately 1 cm apart within the muscle.

5.4.2 Temporalis

A dilution of 5 U per 0.1 mL of onabotulinumtoxinA is used for the temporalis muscle. The muscle belly and temporal line are palpated while the patient clenches his or her teeth. The needle is placed through the skin overlying the temporalis muscle and position is confirmed with the brisk EMG activity that occurs with the patient's teeth clenching. To enhance the accuracy of the injection into the thin temporalis muscle, the needle is usually inserted along the anterior or superior border of the temporalis muscle, and subsequently advanced posteriorly or inferiorly in the sagittal plane, once the correct depth of the needle placement is confirmed with the EMG (▶ Fig. 5.9). This allows multiple aliquots to be injected with one pass of the needle, a technique that is impossible if the needle is passed in a lateral to medial direction. Using the previously described technique, 0.1 mL aliquots are delivered at four or five points within the temporalis muscle. These aliquots are spaced at 1-cm intervals, preferably through one to three skin puncture sites.

5.4.3 Anterior Digastric Belly

A dilution of 5 U per 0.1 mL of onabotulinumtoxinA is used. The neck is extended and the patient is asked to open the jaw widely to allow palpation of the anterior digastric muscle belly. The needle is placed through the skin into the muscle

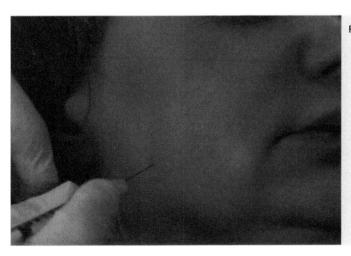

Fig. 5.8 Masseter muscle injection.

closer to the mentum than to the hyoid to minimize dysphagia. Position is confirmed by brisk EMG activity on mouth opening, and 0.1 mL aliquots are injected at multiple sites. The procedure is repeated on the contralateral side.

5.4.4 External Pterygoid

There are two approaches for the treatment of the external or lateral pterygoid muscle. The extraoral cutaneous approach is introduced between the two heads of the mandible. Because this approach is perpendicular to the muscle, it can be less reliable and does not allow for multiple injection points. The intraoral approach allows for better distribution of the toxin along the muscle (▶ Fig. 5.10).

The clinician uses a headlight for intraoral visualization, and the patient is asked to open the mouth fully. The clinician's index finger is used to retract the cheek laterally, and then the patient is asked to close the mouth just slightly while the external pterygoid plate is palpated posterolateral to the last upper molar and medial to the ramus of the mandible. The needle is angled approximately 20 degrees superiorly and laterally and advanced in the long axis of the muscle. Correct placement is confirmed by asking the patient to move the jaw side to side until sharp EMG activity is heard.

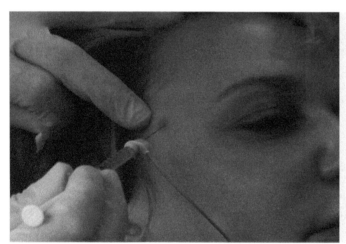

Fig. 5.9 Temporalis muscle injection.

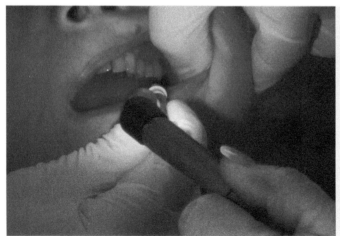

Fig. 5.10 External pterygoid muscle injection.

OnabotulinumtoxinA is injected at two or three points along this axis, advancing the needle and confirming the position in the muscle with EMG recruitment prior to each injection. The same procedure is repeated on the contralateral side. Dosing starts at 10 U of onabotulinumtoxinA per muscle and can be altered according to treatment response. For an asymmetric jaw swing, differential dosing can be employed with an extra 5 to 10 U given in the more active muscle (opposite to the direction of jaw swing).

5.4.5 Internal Pterygoid

The internal or medial pterygoid is not routinely injected as a first-line muscle for OMD but rather is added to the treatment regimen for patients with an inadequate response. OnabotulinumtoxinA is diluted to 5 U per 0.1 mL. The needle is placed through the skin in the submandibular area and directed superiorly deep to the mandible and the U-shaped sling,

which the masseter forms with the internal pterygoid, and along the inner aspect of the mandibular ramus, thus entering the muscle (▶ Fig. 5.11). The position is confirmed by brisk EMG activity when the patient is asked to clench, and the muscle is injected at two to three points. The same procedure is performed on the contralateral side. Rarely, the facial artery, internal maxillary artery, or arterial branches may be encountered during these injections.

5.4.6 Dosing

The clinician's approach to target muscles and dosing of patients with OMD should be based on the specific characteristics and nuance of the involved movements. Specific onabotulinumtoxinA dosing protocols have been established based on published series of OMD patients. Treatment is equal and bilateral in most cases; however, asymmetric dosing may be more prevalent in

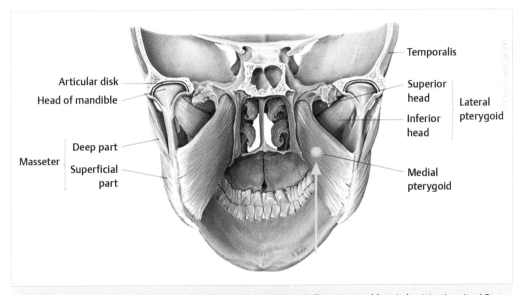

Fig. 5.11 Internal pterygoid muscle injection. Blue arrow = injection needle trajectory; blue circle = injection site. (From Gilroy AM et al. Atlas of Anatomy. 1st Ed. New York: Thieme Medical Publishers; 2008. Based on: Schuenke M, Schulte E, Schumacher U. THIEME Atlas of Anatomy: Head and Neuroanatomy. Illustrations by Voll M and Wesker K. 1st Ed. New York: Thieme Medical Publishers; 2008.)

jaw-deviation management. The below dosing regimens are adapted from these series from Gonzalez-Alegre et al and Sinclair et al.[6,8]

Dosage for Jaw-Closing OMD

Initiate dosing at 20 to 30 U onabotulinumtoxinA to each masseter muscle with an optional 15 to 25 U to each temporalis muscle. The external pterygoid can be treated with 7.5 U if jaw deviation is present. If there is no response, then the aforementioned dosages may be doubled and an additional 10 U may be added to the internal pterygoid muscle. If there is partial response, then an additional 5 to 10 U added to each masseter muscle, optional 5 to 10 U to each temporalis muscle and 10 U should be added to each internal pterygoid muscle.[6,8]

Dosage for Jaw-Opening OMD

Treatment begins with 7.5 to 10 U onabotulinumtoxinA to each external pterygoid and/or 5 U to each anterior belly digastric muscle. If jaw deviation is present, the anterior aspect of the temporalis muscles may be injected with 15 to 25 U. If platysma is involved, then 7.5 U may be injected to each side. Nonresponders should be treated with double initial dose, adding the anterior belly digastric if it was not included in initial treatment. Partial responders may require 5 to 10 U additional to the external pterygoid muscles.[6,8]

Dosage for Lateral Jaw-Deviation OMD

Initial management is composed of 7.5 U injected to the external pterygoid with the optional 15 to 25 U injected to the anterior aspect of the temporalis muscles. Nonresponders should be treated with double the dose to external pterygoids

and add the temporalis treatment if not included at initial injection. Partial responders should receive additional 2.5 to 10 U per external pterygoid muscle. Some patients will demonstrate unilateral tendencies of the jaw deviation. These patients may benefit from asymmetric dosing: higher dose should be delivered to the contralateral external pterygoid and the ipsilateral temporalis muscles.[8]

5.5 Follow-up

The response to the initial treatment is monitored by clinical assessment at the 3- to 4-week mark. Patients are questioned about persistent symptoms and side effects. Repeat observation facilitates targeting muscle groups that need further treatment. Asymmetric movements are also assessed at this point, and some muscle groups may require further unilateral treatment. The dosing of follow-up treatments is assessed individually but typically is lower than that of the initial treatment. Subsequent treatments are at the patient's discretion; the average patient returns every 3 to 4 months. Dosing is adjusted according to the side-effect profile and the length of effect, and the patient is asked to call 3 weeks after the treatment to report any side effects, undesired effects, or inadequate response.

5.6 Complications and Pitfalls

Patients are extensively counseled prior to treatment about the potential risks of excessive toxin dosing, inaccurate needle placement, or toxin diffusion. The most common side effect is weakness of mastication. Long-term side effects of treatment may include temporalis and masseter hypofunctional atrophy with associated changes in facial morphology.

Rare complications due to inaccurate needle placement or toxin diffusion include dysphagia and dysarthria (hyoid and tongue musculature), velopharyngeal incompetence or perioral incompetence, and facial asymmetry (facial musculature). These are always self-limiting and they resolve within 3 months, but may have significant impact on the patient's quality of life. Development of severe dysphagia is a risk[15] and may require feeding with a nasogastric tube until the effects of the treatment subside.

5.7 Conclusion

Oromandibular dystonia can involve isolated or multiple muscle groups of the face and neck. The dystonic contractions often cause functional and social challenges to the patients. Treatment with BoNT can help alleviate the hyperfunctional contractions and improve the individual's quality of life.[16,17,18] Given the complex, dynamic oromandibular musculature, which is involved in chewing and speaking, the treatment of these muscles can often adversely affect the desired normal function of the target muscle groups. Successful treatment often hinges upon selectively treating the most affected muscles and titrating the dose of BoNT for the greatest benefit with the least amount of undesired or adverse effects. Complementary management with oral medications often ameliorates the overall symptomatology.

5.8 Key Points/Pearls

- Oromandibular dystonia (OMD) affects various muscles and muscle groups of the face, mouth, head, and neck.
- OMD is a neurological diagnosis related to basal ganglia or cerebellar dysfunction.

- Jaw-closing OMD responds better than other types of OMD to botulinum toxin injections.
- BoNT injections are an effective local treatment.
- Adverse effects of BoNT injections include masticator fatigue, tongue hypomobility, velopharyngeal incompetence, perioral incompetence.

Oromandibular Dystonia

Most oromandibular dystonia (OMD) is related to closing symptoms. The injection of the masseter and temporalis muscles can be seen in **Video 12.1**. The opening type of OMD is usually treated with injections of the external pterygoid muscles, also seen in **Video 12.1**. Occasionally, the anterior belly of the digastric muscles is injected under the mentum close to the chin, to prevent diffusion to the tongue base and consequent dysphagia.

References

[1] Druckman R, Seelinger D, Thulin B. Chronic involuntary movements induced by phenothiazines. J Nerv Ment Dis.; 135:69–76

[2] Sankhla C, Lai EC, Jankovic J. Peripherally induced oromandibular dystonia. J Neurol Neurosurg Psychiatry.; 65(5): 722–728

[3] Thorburn DN, Lee KH. Oromandibular dystonia following dental treatment: case reports and discussion. N Z Dent J.; 105(1): 18–21

[4] Neychev VK, Fan X, Mitev VI, Hess EJ, Jinnah HA. The basal ganglia and cerebellum interact in the expression of dystonic movement. Brain.; 131(Pt 9):2499–2509

[5] Weiner WJ, Nora LM. "Trick" movements in facial dystonia. J Clin Psychiatry.; 45(12):519–521

[6] Gonzalez-Alegre P, Schneider RL, Hoffman H. Clinical, etiological, and therapeutic features of jaw-opening and jaw-closing oromandibular dystonias: A decade of experience at a single treatment center. Tremor Other Hyperkinet Mov (N Y).; 4:231

[7] Yoshida K. Sensory trick splint as a multimodal therapy for oromandibular dystonia. J Prosthodont Res.; 62(2):239–244

[8] Sinclair CF, Gurey LE, Blitzer A. Oromandibular dystonia: long-term management with botulinum toxin. Laryngoscope.; 123(12):3078–3083

[9] Brin MF, Fahn S, Moskowitz C, et al. Localized injections of botulinum toxin for the treatment of focal dystonia and hemifacial spasm. Mov Disord.; 2(4):237–254

[10] Blitzer A, Brin MF, Greene PE, Fahn S. Botulinum toxin injection for the treatment of oromandibular dystonia. Ann Otol Rhinol Laryngol.; 98(2):93–97

[11] Van Eijden TM, Korfage JA, Brugman P. Architecture of the human jaw-closing and jaw-opening muscles. Anat Rec.; 248 (3):464–474

[12] Tan EK, Jankovic J. Botulinum toxin A in patients with oromandibular dystonia: long-term follow-up. Neurology.; 53(9):2102–2107

[13] Charles PD, Davis TL, Shannon KM, Hook MA, Warner JS. Tongue protrusion dystonia: treatment with botulinum toxin. South Med J.; 90(5):522–525

[14] Esper CD, Freeman A, Factor SA. Lingual protrusion dystonia: frequency, etiology and botulinum toxin therapy. Parkinsonism Relat Disord.; 16(7):438–441

[15] Hermanowicz N, Truong DD. Treatment of oromandibular dystonia with botulinum toxin. Laryngoscope.; 101(11): 1216–1218

[16] Scorr LM, Silver MR, Hanfelt J, et al. Pilot single-blind trial of abobotulinumtoxinA in oromandibular dystonia. Neurotherapeutics.; 15(2):452–458

[17] Charous SJ, Comella CL, Fan W. Jaw-opening dystonia: quality of life after botulinum toxin injections. Ear Nose Throat J.; 90(2):E9

[18] Teemul TA, Patel R, Kanatas A, Carter LM. Management of oromandibular dystonia with botulinum A toxin: a series of cases. Br J Oral Maxillofac Surg.; 54(10):1080–1084

6
Botulinum Neurotoxin for Spasmodic Dysphonia

Phillip C. Song, Lucian Sulica, and Andrew Blitzer

Summary

Botulinum neurotoxin (BoNT) injection into the larynx for symptomatic control of spasmodic dysphonia has been in use for over three decades and has been the gold standard of treatment for most of that time, endorsed as primary therapy by the American Academy of Otolaryngology–Head and Neck Surgery (Policy Statement: Botulinum Toxin; reaffirmed March 1, 1999). This chapter reviews the options for diagnosis and treatment of spasmodic dysphonia, with particular attention to treatment with BoNT.

Keywords: adductor spasmodic dysphonia, abductor spasmodic dysphonia, laryngeal spasm, laryngeal dystonia, laryngeal electromyography, botulinum toxin treatment

6.1 Introduction

Spasmodic dysphonia is a clinical syndrome characterized by involuntary, hyperfunctional spasms or postures of the intrinsic laryngeal musculature, yielding abnormal speech. Traube[1] first used the term *spastic dysphonia* to describe patients with nervous hoarseness in 1871. Historically, the terms *mogiphonia, spastic dysphonia, aspartic aphonia, phonic laryngeal spasm,* and *coordinated laryngeal spasm* have been used to describe the same clinical presentation.[2,3] Long thought to be psychological, spasmodic dysphonia was shown to be clearly organic and neurologic in nature by the dramatic response to nerve section in pioneering work by Dedo and Behlau.[4] In 1982, Marsden and Sheehy[5] proposed that spasmodic dysphonia represented a laryngeal dystonia. They noted that "all evidence points to the conclusion that blepharospasm and oromandibular dystonia seen in Meige [syndrome] is another manifestation of adult onset torsion dystonia, [and] since dysphonia may occur in the same syndrome, it is quite likely that dysphonia itself may be the sole manifestation of dystonia." In 1988, Blitzer and colleagues[6] showed through clinical examination and laryngeal electromyography (EMG) that features of spastic dysphonia were entirely consistent with focal cranial dystonia. With growing advances in brain mapping and neurogenetics, the neurological underpinnings of spasmodic dysphonia and other laryngeal dystonias are being discovered.[7] Functional magnetic resonance imaging (MRI) has showed changes in the corticobulbar tracts connecting motor sensory centers within the cortex to phonatory motoneurons in the brainstem[8] and genetic screening continues to provide connections between laryngeal dystonias and other neurological diseases.

6.2 Classification and Presentation

Spasmodic dysphonia is classified as a laryngeal dystonia, a clinical term used to describe an action-induced, task-specific, laryngeal neuromuscular disorder resulting in disturbance in the production of connected speech.[9] Dystonias are classified by clinical symptom, age at onset, distribution, and cause. When classified by distribution, dystonias are categorized as focal, segmental, multifocal, or generalized. Spasmodic dysphonia is a focal dystonia involving the laryngeal adductor muscles (lateral cricoarytenoid, interarytenoid, thyroarytenoid, and possibly the cricothyroid), abductor muscles (posterior cricoarytenoid [PCA]), or both, with occasional involvement of supraglottic structures. The degree and topography of laryngeal muscle involvement appears to vary, and the clinical manifestation may actually represent the predominant activity rather than pure, mutually exclusive adductor or abductor muscle involvement.[10] Laryngeal dystonia may also affect other functions of the larynx besides connected speech. Both singer's dystonia and respiratory adductor dystonia have been described.[11,12]

The majority of dystonias are primary, or of idiopathic etiology, although as many as a third of patients identify a precipitating factor or incident.[13] These patients have a normal perinatal and early developmental history; no prior history of head trauma or neurologic illness; no exposure to drugs known to cause acquired dystonia (e.g., phenothiazines); and normal intellectual, pyramidal, cerebellar, and sensory examinations. Identification of any cause by such history, examination, or laboratory studies defines secondary dystonia. Most cases of spasmodic dysphonia have no manifestations outside of the larynx, consistent with their identifications a focal dystonias. Rarely, cases may be associated with or progress to symptoms in another part of the body. Although in our experience this is a very small percentage, rates as high as 17% have been reported.[7] Multiple factors have been noted to cause secondary laryngeal dystonia. These may include neurologic disorders, drug exposures, and Parkinsonism.

Clinically, spasmodic dysphonia is divided into abductor, adductor dysphonia, "singer's dysphonia," and adductor respiratory dystonia. In adductor spasmodic dysphonia, patients present with a choked, strain-strangled voice, breaks in phonation, diminished volume, and a monotonal pitch. Patients with the abductor type present with a breathy, effortful voice, abrupt breaks in fluency, and whispered elements of speech. With severe spasms, patients may be aphonic. Compensatory behaviors may mask the patient's true voice pattern. Patients with a severe adductor spasmodic dysphonia may exhibit compensatory abductor voicing, with aphonia or whispering.[14] Although some authors believe that all patients with spasmodic dysphonia have abductor and adductor involvement, with symptoms manifesting according to the predominant type,[15,16] the main premise of botulinum toxin treatment, chemodenervation of the hyperfunctional muscle group, is well served by the adductor–abductor classification.

In both groups, patients may demonstrate a phonation-associated tremor. In contrast to essential tremor, the spasmodic dysphonia–associated tremor is irregular and may be secondary to posturing of dystonic muscles in a position in which the agonist contractions do not fully neutralize those of the antagonist muscles. Blitzer and colleagues[17] showed that 25% of spasmodic dysphonia patients may have such a tremor. Distinguishing dystonic tremor from essential voice tremor may occasionally be exceptionally challenging.

6.3 Diagnosis and Investigation

The diagnosis of spasmodic dysphonia is clinical, based principally on perceptual analysis of the voice, complemented by the laryngoscopic examination. Evaluation should include a detailed head and neck and neurologic examination, with particular attention paid to spasm, dysfunction, or tremor in any area of the head and neck. Laryngoscopy should be performed with flexible transnasal instrumentation, because it disrupts physiologic laryngeal function least, and allows assessment of connected speech as well as swallowing and breathing. The rigid telescope may have a role for the detailed evaluation of the vibratory margin of the vocal fold, and to exclude mucosal wave pathology, but is likely to obscure the tell-tale signs of spasmodic dysphonia. The nuances of diagnosis are beyond the scope of this chapter, but the primary diagnostic challenge is differentiating between spasmodic dysphonia, muscle tension dysphonia (MTD), and vocal tremor, or combinations of the three. Leonard and Kendall[18] noted that motion abnormalities in spasmodic dysphonia were present only during specific speaking actions, whereas they were present more consistently during MTD and vocal tremor.

Identification of intermittent hyperfunctional breaks and spasms, with excessive and inappropriate adduction or abduction of the vocal folds during specific vocal tasks, is the basis for the diagnosis of spasmodic dysphonia. The spasms and breaks have a characteristic and reproducible pattern that can be elicited using a standardized set of sentences. During the endoscopic laryngeal exam, adductor-type spasmodic dysphonia typically demonstrates intermittent, occasionally more sustained, hyperadductory postures with hyperfunctional closure of at least the true and sometimes the false vocal folds, excessive medial rotation of the vocalis process, or excessive vocal fold tension that corresponds to the choked, strained-strangled voice breaks. Adductor spasms typically occur with voiced onsets. The laryngeal exam for abductor-type spasmodic dysphonia should exhibit inappropriate abduction during connected speech, which results in a breathy, although effortful, voice quality with aphonic or whispered segments. Abductor spasms are marked when trying to phonate a vowel after a voiceless consonant (example /h/, /p/, or /t/), in contrast to other causes of breathy voice from glottic insufficiency such as vocal fold paralysis or presbylarynges, which yield a more consistent breathy quality to the voice. The presence of secondary functional or compensatory postures may render the diagnosis difficult, and a short course of voice therapy may be useful to identify and address these.

Ludlow and colleagues emphasized the need for a standardized diagnostic criterion to help differentiate between vocal tremor, MTD, and spasmodic dysphonia[19] and proposed a three-tier system for the diagnosis of spasmodic dysphonia. Tier one is a screening questionnaire that consists of four questions (▶ Table 6.1).

Patients are expected to have had symptoms for at least 3 months and answer in the affirmative to the first two questions to be considered as having possible spasmodic dysphonia. Tier two is a clinical speech examination in which patients are taken through a series of vocal exercises by a voice specialist. Specific sentences are used to elicit abductor and adductor voice breaks. Patients are expected to have one or voice

Table 6.1 Screening questions for spasmodic dysphonia

Question	Usually expected for spasmodic dysphonia	Not expected for spasmodic dysphonia
1. Does it take a lot of work for you to talk?	Yes	No
2. Is it sometimes easier and sometimes more difficult to talk?	Yes	Sometimes normal without treatment
3. How long has it been difficult for you to talk?	3 mos or more, a chronic problem	Less than 3 mo
4. Can you do any of the following normally?		
Shout	Yes	No
Cry	Yes	No
Laugh	Yes	No
Whisper	Yes	Same as speech
Sing	Yes	More affected than speech
Yawn	Yes	No

Source: Data from Ludlow CL, Naunton RF, Fujita M, Sedory SE. Spasmodic dysphonia: botulinum toxin injection after recurrent nerve surgery. Otolaryngol Head Neck Surg 1990;102:122–131.

breaks during speaking and fewer during whispering to be included. Tier three, fiberoptic laryngoscopy, reveals normal glottal function with swallowing, whistling, and coughing while demonstrating vocal fold spasm, or tremor while speaking sentences. Using this three-tiered technique on a series of 30 patients with known MTD, spasmodic dysphonia, or tremor, Ludlow and colleagues[20] were able to correctly categorize 97% of patients.

Objective testing and other diagnostic modalities can be useful in the diagnosis of difficult cases. In assessing the utility of acoustic analysis, Zwirner and coworkers[21] found significantly higher mean values of standard deviation of fundamental frequency, jitter, shimmer, and voice break factor, and significantly lower mean values of signal-to-noise ratio in spasmodic dysphonia patients when compared with normal controls.

Using acoustic analysis, Sapienza and coworkers[22] found that only patients with adductor spasmodic dysphonia manifested voice breaks during speech, specifically with sustained vowels. They also found patients with adductor spasmodic dysphonia to have greater variation in the type of acoustic event produced as a function of speech task. Koufman[23] found spectral analysis to be useful in differentiating adductor spasmodic dysphonia and MTD, sometimes a challenging task given the supraglottic hyperfunction that may be present in both processes. Koufman noted that voice breaks were usually present in spasmodic dysphonia but absent in MTD. The spasmodic dysphonia patients also had well-defined formants, whereas the MTD patients did not, and the MTD patients had excessive high-frequency spectral noise that was minimal in spasmodic dysphonia patients.[23] This showed that spectral analysis, although not a frequently used tool, may be a useful adjunct to differentiate adductor spasmodic dysphonia from MTD.

Typically, laryngeal EMG demonstrates abnormal, but not pathognomonic, findings. Large and polyphasic motor unit potentials and an abnormally long latency from the initiation of electrical signal to the beginning of sound production have been reported.[24,25] Nash and Ludlow[26,27] compared laryngeal EMG results in patients with adductor spasmodic dysphonia against controls. They found a significant increase in mean muscle activity during voice breaks in the thyroarytenoid muscle, unsurprising given the phenomenology of the disorder, whereas muscle tone in these patients was equivalent to controls during normal speech. Hillel[10] found abnormal laryngeal EMG patterns of response, increased latencies, and increased amplitudes of recruitment in many tasks including nonphonatory tasks among all spasmodic dysphonia patients. Most importantly, his work revealed demonstrated abnormal activity in all five intrinsic laryngeal muscles and previously undocumented variability in muscle involvement, revealing more complexity in the disease than commonly assumed.

About 12 to 15% of patients with spasmodic dysphonia have a positive family history and genetic testing shows promise as a diagnostic modality. Several genes have been associated with laryngeal dystonias. Notable gene regions and mutations that have laryngeal dystonia as a manifestation include TOR1A (DYT1), TAF1 (DYT4), THAP 1 (DYT6), and GNAL (DYT25). Most of these genes are associated with regional manifestations of dystonia or other neurological features such as Parkinsonism. At this point, however, routine genetic testing for isolated laryngeal dystonia has a low yield, but in the context of other neurological symptoms family history can be considered.[28]

Functional MRI features for laryngeal dystonia are quickly evolving and alterations in brain connections are being described with more specificity in spasmodic dysphonia. Functional MRI can show metabolic activity during tasks such as vocalization. Changes in the connectivity between different regions associated with voice tasks have been demonstrated in patients with spasmodic dysphonia.[29]

The diagnosis of spasmodic dysphonia can be made reliably with the patient's history and physical examination. Acoustic analysis and laryngeal EMG both have shown promise as aids for difficult cases, but more research is required to better define their role. The cornerstone of diagnosis at this time remains a carefully directed history with appropriate screening questions, speech examination, and flexible laryngoscopy.

6.4 Treatment

Botulinum neurotoxin type A injections into the intrinsic laryngeal muscles represent the current standard for the treatment of spasmodic dysphonia. There have been hundreds of peer-reviewed articles investigating the utility of BoNT injections for spasmodic dysphonia, with the collective evidence overwhelmingly favoring the effectiveness of this modality.

In 2015, Blitzer et al updated their experience of BoNT treatment for spasmodic dysphonia.[30] They found that 90% of patients improved for 3 to 12 months after injection of BoNT-A, with a need for repeat injections every 3 to 6 months. Two meta-analyses have been performed that considered the efficacy of BoNT, and one blinded, randomized controlled trial has been conducted in which BoNT injection was compared with saline injection and measured with objective acoustic outcomes.[31,32,33] BoNT-A markedly reduced perturbation, decreased fundamental frequency range, and improved spectrographic characteristics.

Although the main effect of BoNT is a blockade of the injected muscle at the neuromuscular junction in the peripheral nervous system, this explanation does not seem to correlate with the pathophysiologic model of spasmodic dysphonia or the surprising efficacy of this injection, suggesting an effect on the central nervous system. Byrnes and colleagues[34] showed that BoNT injections caused a transient change in the mapping of muscle representation areas in the motor cortex. This has further been suggested by the effect of BoNT on noninjected laryngeal muscles in spasmodic dysphonia.[35] In 2007, Antonucci et al[36] demonstrated that BoNT is translocated to the afferent synapses in the contralateral hemisphere in mice and rats. Although these mechanisms are not completely understood, the efficacy and safety of BoNT have led to its being deemed the primary therapy for spasmodic dysphonia.

The target muscle for BoNT injection depends on the relative adductor and abductor features of the spasmodic dysphonia. The standard treatment for adductor spasmodic dysphonia at the majority of voice centers is bilateral EMG-guided transcutaneous injections into the thyroarytenoid muscle, using equal amounts of BoNT; however, there are several variations of this approach. The dose of BoNT given, the time course between injections, unilateral versus bilateral injections, and the follow-up can vary between centers and among individual practitioners. In addition, there seems to be great variability in the BoNT sensitivity and recovery among patients as well as fluctuations in the disease symptoms. In essence, each patient requires an individualized plan of care, and practitioners may need to alter their injection methods, doses, and schedules accordingly to maximize efficacy.

The efficacy of bilateral thyroarytenoid injections has been the most studied and has the most robust and longest treatment history. However, some small studies have shown that unilateral injections may have equivalent improvement in voice symptoms and sometimes improved therapeutic profiles.[37,38,39] Adams and colleagues[37] compared 15 patients receiving a 15-unit (U) unilateral injection of BoNT with 11 patients receiving bilateral 2.5-U injections. They found that both the unilateral and bilateral BoNT injections were associated with significant improvements in spasmodic dysphonia, and both types of injections were associated with a significant increase in vocal breathiness at 2 weeks postinjection. However, in using acoustic analysis to compare the two, they found

that maximum phonation time, vocal jitter, and the number of voice breaks per second indicated that unilateral BoNT injections may provide superior and longer lasting benefits than bilateral BoNT injections. The same group again compared unilateral and bilateral injections in 1995, treating 25 patients with a 15-U unilateral injection and 25 patients with bilateral 2.5-U injections. They found comparable results at 2 and 6 weeks using acoustic analysis. However, the bilateral group was noted to have a significant reduction in maximum phonation time in comparison with the unilateral group.[38] Upile and colleagues[39] examined 31 patients with adductor spasmodic dysphonia who received either unilateral or bilateral injections. They found that bilateral injections were associated with postinjection voice loss, whereas unilateral injections were not.

Ford et al[40] described indirect laryngoscopy for guidance in performing thyroarytenoid injections. In their study, a slightly delayed time of onset was noted. However, the efficacy and duration of the injections were not significantly changed from the standard EMG-guided injections. They pointed out that although most otolaryngologists are unfamiliar with laryngeal EMG, most are comfortable with laryngoscopy. Flexible laryngoscopy has been used both to visualize percutaneous thyroarytenoid injection and to guide injections through the channel of the laryngoscope.[41,42,43] Although perhaps more familiar, these approaches have limitations. Transoral injection may be limited or made impossible by the patient's gag reflex. Injection through a flexible bronchoscopic needle entails waste of BoNT to fill the needle tubing and makes precision difficult to control.[9] The aforementioned techniques also do not allow for EMG confirmation of needle placement, which allows for controlled administration of treatment into the more actively contracting regions of the muscle, near motor end-plates and the site of BoNT action.

Injection of the thyroarytenoid muscles may be used for adductor spasmodic dysphonia in patients with previous recurrent laryngeal nerve section.[44] Analysis of treatment results in this population suggests that injection of muscles on the side of the previous nerve section tends to optimize results and minimize adverse effects.[45] Ludlow and colleagues[46] reported a significant reduction in all speech symptoms using bilateral thyroarytenoid injections in the setting of previous recurrent laryngeal nerve section.

In patients with abductor spasmodic dysphonia, the target muscles for denervation are the PCA muscles. In our practice, these injections are generally not performed simultaneously to minimize airway risk from impaired abduction. The larynx is reexamined 2 weeks postinjection to determine the therapeutic effect and airway patency, and plan the contralateral injection, usually at half the initial dose. Using this technique, Blitzer et al[47] noted that patients achieved 70.3% of normal voice. In other centers, bilateral simultaneous injections may be the norm: simultaneous injections have been shown to be reasonably safe by Stong and colleagues,[48] who performed a series of simultaneous bilateral PCA injections without airway complications.

The interarytenoid muscle was found to be dysfunctional in certain cases by Hillel and colleagues[49] using five-lead EMG. They found that the interarytenoid muscle can be injected in conjunction with the thyroarytenoid muscle to treat certain cases of refractory spasmodic dysphonia.

6.5 Other Treatments

Systemic medications may help reduce symptoms and may work in conjunction with BoNT injections to prolong the therapeutic effect. The most common medications for the treatment of dystonia are oral anticholinergics. However, the side-effect profiles for these medications are broad and include difficulty with concentration, cognitive impairment, dry mouth, urinary retention, and blurred vision. Local anticholinesterases can ameliorate some of these side effects. Baclofen has been found to have the greatest therapeutic effect with the best side-effect profile.[9] In the authors' experience, oral anticholinergics are rarely used for patients with isolated voice symptoms related to spasmodic dysphonia. Sodium oxybate (Xyrem, Jazz Pharmaceuticals, Dublin, Ireland) is an GABAergic medication used for cataplexy and narcolepsy which has shown efficacy for voice improvement in an open label trial.[50]

Surgical management of spasmodic dysphonia remains a controversial area with a chequered history. Spasmodic dysphonia owes its identification as a neurologic disease to initial positive results of nerve section; Dedo and Behlau, who initially conceived and executed the operation, reported an 85% success rate after unilateral recurrent laryngeal nerve section.[4] However, subsequent reports revealed a high rate of symptom recurrence after months to years.[51] Several surgical techniques, including recurrent laryngeal nerve avulsion, laryngeal framework surgery, partial and total laser thyroarytenoid muscle resection, implantable stimulators, and selective laryngeal adductor denervation–reinnervation using the ansa cervicalis, have been used to circumvent the problem of long-term failure with inconsistent success.[52,53,54,55,56] Prolonged or permanent breathiness, unilateral vocal fold paralysis, dyskinesis and synkinesis, as well as recurrence of symptoms have prevented surgery from being a primary modality for treatment. A recent poll on patients who underwent selective laryngeal adductor denervation–reinnervation surgery reported that 82% of the patients would recommend the procedure to others (whereas 18% would not) but also noted 31% had postoperative dysphagia. A recent comparative analysis of BoNT injections versus surgery suggests that both interventions have reported benefits.[57,58]

6.6 Injection Technique

Our method for laryngeal muscle injection does not require an endoscope or an assistant. We use a 27-gauge insulated needle attached to an EMG, functioning like a monopolar electrode. A standard dilution of 4.0 mL of sterile saline/100-U vial of BoNT (Botox, Allergan plc, Irvine, CA) results in a concentration of 2.5 mouse units per 0.1 mL which can be further diluted as necessary for each patient to deliver the appropriate dose in a typical volume of 0.1 mL per vocal fold. For instance, to deliver 1.0 mouse unit to the vocal fold, 0.1 mL of stock solution (2.5 U) is diluted to 0.25 mL, creating a concentration of 1.0 U per 0.1 mL. Limiting injection volume is meant to prevent airway obstruction, as well as unwanted diffusion of the drug. We report below on starting injection doses used at our institutions; however, it should be noted that there is significant variation on starting dosages and schedules among practitioners. Chang et al[59] found that dosage of BoNT-A had a positive correlation with the duration of negative side effects, but a negative correlation with the duration of

the normal voice. They posit that their analysis only witnessed the downward trend of what is likely a bell-curve effect in dosing on the normal voice.

Our experience with BoNT injections in the larynx mostly has been with onabotulinum toxin (Botox, Allergan plc), and therefore most dosing guidelines in this chapter are specific for Botox. Rimabotulinum toxin type B (Myobloc; Solstice Neurosciences Inc., South San Francisco, CA) and abobotulinum toxin type A (Dysport; Medicis Pharmaceutical, Scottsdale, AZ) are available alternatives, but dosing will need to be adjusted. It should be noted that the diffusion characteristics among the three toxins are slightly different, and that rimabotulinum toxin type B has been associated with a potentially higher autonomic effects (dry mouth).

For patients with suspected blocking antibody formation who respond poorly to BoNT-A, BoNT-B (rimabotulinum toxin type B; Myobloc) has been shown to be a safe and effective alternative.[60] Blitzer[61] showed that Myobloc is effective at a dose ratio of roughly 52 U/1 U, and has a more rapid onset of action but a shorter duration.

6.6.1 Adductor Spasmodic Dysphonia

The thyroarytenoid muscle, targeted in the treatment of adductor spasmodic dysphonia, arises from the inner surface of the angle of the thyroid cartilage and cricothyroid ligament and inserts on the anterolateral surface of the arytenoid cartilage. The inferomedial fibers of the thyroarytenoid muscle are known as the vocalis muscle (▶ Fig. 6.1). The proximity of the thyroarytenoid muscle to the cricothyroid membrane allows for injection of the muscle through the cricothyroid space (▶ Fig. 6.2, ▶ Fig. 6.3).

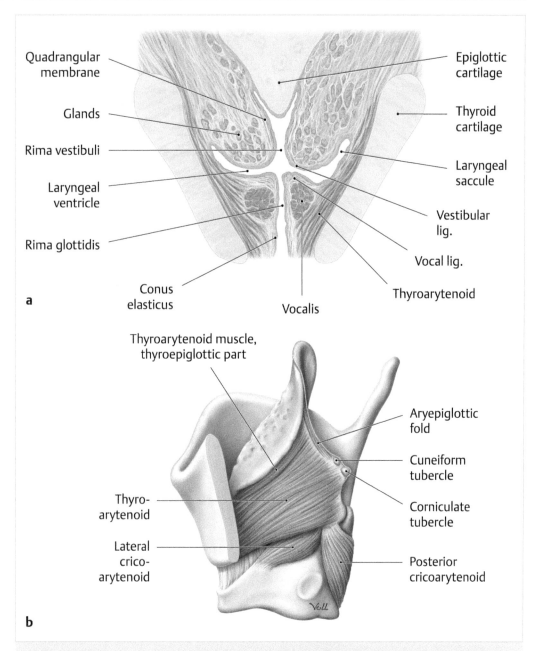

Fig. 6.1 (a,b) Vocal fold anatomy. (From Gilroy AM et al. Atlas of Anatomy. 3rd Ed. New York: Thieme Medical Publishers; 2016. Based on: Schuenke M, Schulte E, Schumacher U. THIEME Atlas of Anatomy: Head and Neuroanatomy. Illustrations by Voll M and Wesker K. 1st Ed. New York: Thieme Medical Publishers; 2008.)

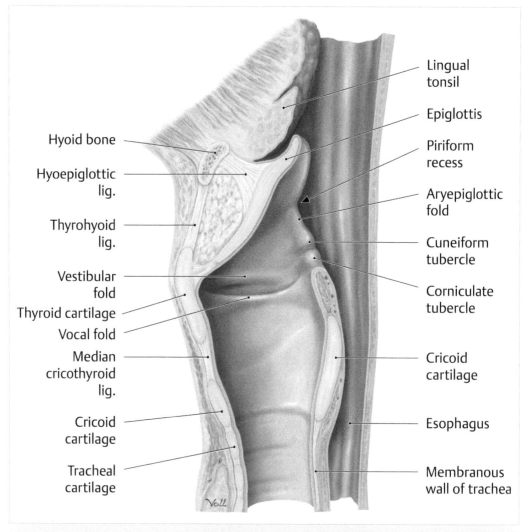

Fig. 6.2 Midsagittal section of larynx. (From Gilroy AM et al. Atlas of Anatomy. 3rd Ed. New York: Thieme Medical Publishers; 2016. Based on: Schuenke M, Schulte E, Schumacher U. THIEME Atlas of Anatomy: Head and Neuroanatomy. Illustrations by Voll M and Wesker K. 1st Ed. New York: Thieme Medical Publishers; 2008.)

The patient is placed in a supine position or beach chair position with the neck gently extended. The patient may also be placed in an upright sitting position with the head in neutral position. The thyroid and cricoid cartilages are identified by palpation, delineating the cricothyroid membrane. The needle is bent superiorly 30 to 45 degrees, and then placed through the cricothyroid membrane in or just off of the midline. It is advanced superiorly and laterally. As the surgeon advances the needle, he or she listens for the muscle interference pattern from the EMG. At this point, a characteristic "buzz" on the EMG indicates that the needle is within the laryngeal air column between the two vocal folds, which means that the needle needs to be redirected laterally. Crossing the endolaryngeal mucosa can irritate the patient, triggering a cough reflex. If the needle is redirected slightly lateral to pierce the cricothyroid membrane a few millimeters off the midline, the needle can be

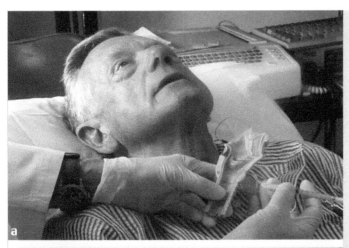

Fig. 6.3 (a,b) Transcricothyroid thyroarytenoid injection technique.

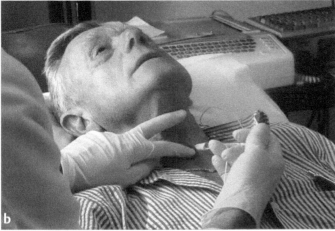

directed into the thyroarytenoid muscle without entering the airway, minimizing the irritation. Once the needle is placed in an area that demonstrates crisp motor unit potentials, placement in the correct muscle is confirmed with a validating maneuver. Asking the patient to say /I/ should result in EMG activation of adductor muscles. The thyroarytenoid muscle will yield sustained activation, whereas the lateral cricoarytenoid will yield a sharp but transient burst of activation concurrent with voice onset. In practice, it is often difficult to direct the needle consistently into one or the other. Happily, the clinical effect does not seem to be compromised as long as one of the adductor muscles is injected. With placement confirmed by EMG, the surgeon then

aspirates to ensure that the needle has not pierced a blood vessel. BoNT is then injected. The authors' typical initial treatment dose is a 1- to 1.25-U injection, and a booster can be given in 2 weeks and titrated to the patient's needs.

6.6.2 Abductor Spasmodic Dysphonia

The PCA is the target muscle for the treatment of abductor spasmodic dysphonia. It arises from the depressions of the posterior aspect of the cricoid lamina. The muscle runs laterally and superiorly to insert onto the posterior aspect of the ipsilateral muscular process of the arytenoid (▶ Fig. 6.4). The position of the PCA

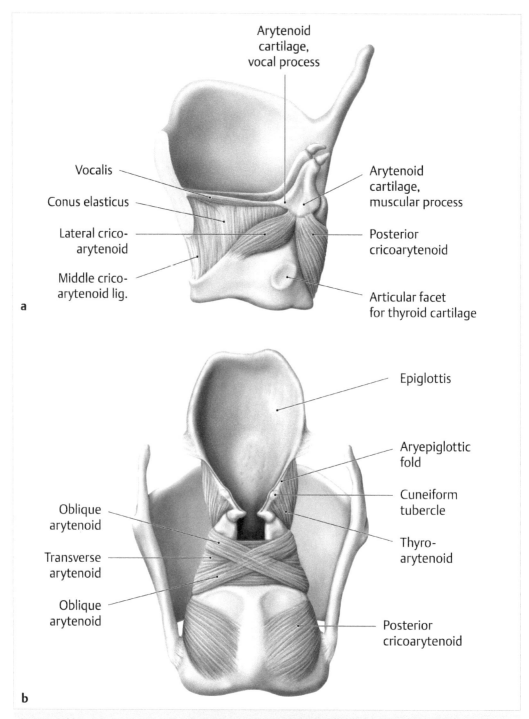

Fig. 6.4 (a,b) Posterior cricoarytenoid muscle anatomy. (From Gilroy AM et al. Atlas of Anatomy. 3rd Ed. New York: Thieme Medical Publishers; 2016. Based on: Schuenke M, Schulte E, Schumacher U. THIEME Atlas of Anatomy: Head and Neuroanatomy. Illustrations by Voll M and Wesker K. 1st Ed. New York: Thieme Medical Publishers; 2008.)

allows for injection in one of two ways. The surgeon may rotate the laryngeal framework laterally for direct access to the posterior aspect of the larynx from the lateral neck, or the surgeon may pass a needle through the cricothyroid membrane, subglottis, and posterior wall of the cricoid cartilage to reach the muscle.

In the laryngeal rotation technique, the patient should be positioned comfortably with the neck and shoulders relaxed to allow for minimal muscle activity. The thumb is placed on the posterior edge of the thyroid cartilage on the side to be injected, with the other four fingers applying gentle pressure on the contralateral thyroid lamina. The larynx is then rotated to expose its posterior aspect. The needle is then inserted along the lower half of the posterior aspect of the thyroid cartilage and advanced until it abuts the hard surface of the cricoid cartilage (▶ Fig. 6.5). It is then pulled back slightly. The validating maneuver in this case consists of a sniff to confirm the position of the needle in the PCA. This method works best on patients with a thin neck and high, mobile larynx.

The transglottic method involves traversing the airway and boring through the cricoid cartilage. The needle is inserted through the cricothyroid membrane in

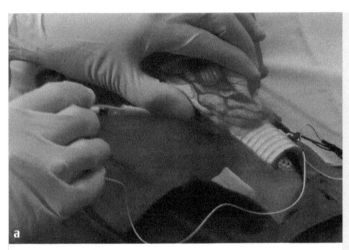
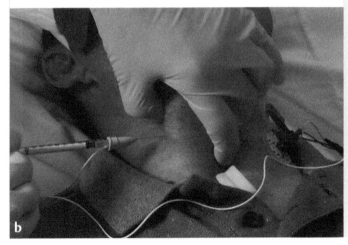

Fig. 6.5 (a,b) Laryngeal rotation posterior cricoarytenoid (PCA) injection technique.

the midline, guided across the subglottic air space, and through the posterior lamina of the cricoid cartilage on one side of the midline or the other (▶ Fig. 6.6, ▶ Fig. 6.7). Generally, with this approach, an intratracheal injection of plain lidocaine is helpful in preventing the patient from coughing. This does not hinder EMG signaling as the target muscle is on the opposite side of the cricoid cartilage from the injection.

Placement is again confirmed by having the patient sniff. This technique is more difficult in older patients, in whom the cartilage may be calcified. In addition, the needle often plugs with cartilage as it transits the cricoid lamina, which may require substantial plunger pressure to clear. Using a syringe with a Luer lock is helpful to prevent separation of the needle in the event. We begin injection with a dose of 3.75 U or 0.15 mL of BoNT to one

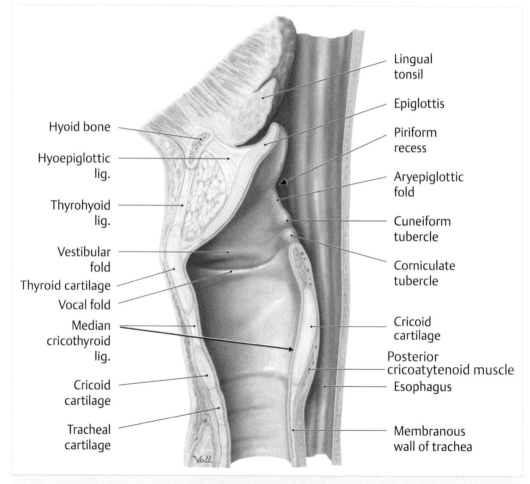

Fig. 6.6 Transglottic posterior cricoarytenoid muscle anatomy. (From Gilroy AM et al. Atlas of Anatomy. 1st Ed. New York: Thieme Medical Publishers; 2008. Based on: Schuenke M, Schulte E, Schumacher U. THIEME Atlas of Anatomy: Head and Neuroanatomy. Illustrations by Voll M and Wesker K. 1st Ed. New York: Thieme Medical Publishers; 2008.)

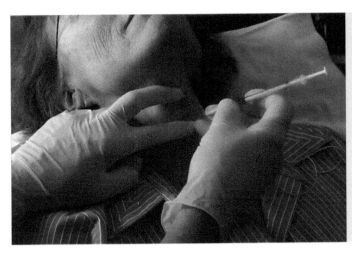

Fig. 6.7 Transglottic posterior cricoarytenoid injection technique.

PCA muscle. The effect this has on the injected muscle is used for dose adjustment 2 weeks later, at the time of injection of the contralateral PCA. In their original investigation of this technique, Blitzer et al[47] found that 19% of patients improved after unilateral injection, and patients on average experienced an overall improvement to 70% of normal function.

6.6.3 Refractory Spasmodic Dysphonia

Some patients do not have a good response to BoNT injections. In these cases, other etiologies of dysphonia should be evaluated. This appears to be more prevalent in abductor spasmodic dysphonia, and is likely due to the fact that the weakness required to control the abductor spasms brings on unacceptable airway symptoms. Some patients develop refractory dysphonic spasms despite a good initial result with toxin injections. Klotz et al[62] demonstrated that multiple different muscles can be involved in refractory spasmodic dysphonia and EMG may be used to show which muscles are involved in a particular case, allowing for better targeting of toxin injections.

Another approach is a trial injection of additional muscle groups. Interarytenoid muscle injection may be performed in patients with adductor spasmodic dysphonia in whom traditional thyroarytenoid injections have not provided relief. Hillel[10] in 2001 initially noted prominent EMG abnormalities of the interarytenoid muscle in patients with adductor spasmodic dysphonia. Hillel et al[49] then studied the effect of interarytenoid BoNT injections in 23 patients. They found a good response in 10 patients, 5 of who had been refractory to traditional BoNT injection. The interarytenoid muscle is the only unpaired intrinsic muscle of the larynx. It is composed of the transverse and oblique portions (▶ Fig. 6.8).

The transverse portion arises from the posterior surface of both arytenoid cartilages, crossing from one to the other. The oblique portion originates from the posterior aspect of the muscular process, crosses the midline, and inserts on the apex of the contralateral arytenoid cartilage. Some fibers continue as the aryepiglottic muscle.[63] The interarytenoid muscle may be approached transglottically, piercing the muscle between the arytenoid towers. It may also be approached through the cricothyroid membrane using laryngeal EMG or direct visualization for guidance.[64] Other potential muscles that have been successfully

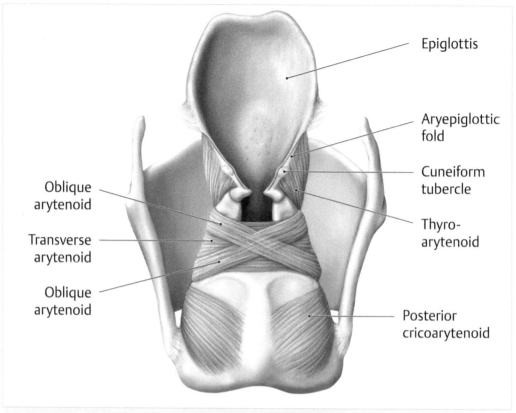

Fig. 6.8 Anatomy of the interarytenoid muscles. (From Gilroy AM et al. Atlas of Anatomy. 3rd Ed. New York: Thieme Medical Publishers; 2016. Based on: Schuenke M, Schulte E, Schumacher U. THIEME Atlas of Anatomy: Head and Neuroanatomy. Illustrations by Voll M and Wesker K. 1st Ed. New York: Thieme Medical Publishers; 2008.)

targeted are the supraglottic musculature in the aryepiglottic fold or the false vocal fold. If patients seem to transition from breathy phonation directly back to hyperfunctional phonation, alternating each vocal fold with larger doses but at shorter intervals may be successful. Finally, if patients seem to lose all response to one serotype of toxin, a different serotype may lead to a good result.

Cricothyroid muscle injections have been used, based on research performed by Ludlow and colleagues,[65] showing abnormal cricothyroid activity in these patients. The cricothyroid muscles are bilateral broad muscles that arise off the lateral aspects of the anterior cricoid and

go lateral and superior toward the lateral thyroid lamina (▶ Fig. 6.9). The needle is inserted along the lateral boundary of the cricothyroid space and is directed superiorly and laterally, staying superficial to the thyroid lamina. When the needle encounters insertional motor activity, the patient is instructed to speak a high-pitched /I/ or perform a pitch glide from the lower register into falsetto. The confirmation is an EMG signal that escalates with higher pitch. The typical starting dose is 3.75 U per side.

Poor treatment results have often been ascribed to the patient's developing antibody-mediated resistance to BoNT-A.[66] This is extremely rare at doses typically

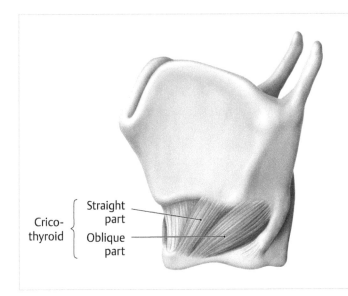

Fig. 6.9 Cricothyroid muscle anatomy. (From Gilroy AM et al. Atlas of Anatomy. 1st Ed. New York: Thieme Medical Publishers; 2008. Based on: Schuenke M, Schulte E, Schumacher U. THIEME Atlas of Anatomy: Head and Neuroanatomy. Illustrations by Voll M and Wesker K. 1st Ed. New York: Thieme Medical Publishers; 2008.)

Crico-thyroid { Straight part / Oblique part

used to treat spasmodic dysphonia. It is our experience that most patients designated as "nonresponders" are simply the recipients of technically poor injections. Injecting BoNT into one half of the patient's frontalis muscle and reassessing activity in 2 weeks is an easy way of proving whether the patient is truly a nonresponder (to both the physician and the patient). Botulinum toxin B is available for the treatment of true nonresponder patients.[60,61]

6.7 Follow-up

Patients are monitored clinically to assess their dose–response. There is a high degree of variability in the dose–response rate and the duration of effect among patients with spasmodic dysphonia. In addition, patient preference and convenience must be taken into account. Patients who cannot attend follow-up easily may require a higher dose of BoNT for the sake of a longer benefit, even though it results temporary breathiness, whereas patients with easy access to the clinic may prefer short-duration, smaller

doses resulting in virtually no breathiness. There is likely a threshold dose after which increased doses increase side effects without providing additional benefit.[59] Some patients with adductor spasmodic dysphonia may also respond better to staggered unilateral doses. Determining optimal dose, distribution and treatment schedule for each patient is a process, made efficient by good feedback from the patient regarding degree and duration of symptom relief, as well as adverse effects, allowing the physician to adjust treatment.

Holden et al[66] retrospectively reviewed a series of 13 adductor spasmodic dysphonia patients, and found that they were able to reach their optimal dose after an average of 2.2 injections. They also found that the patients who started with a dose of 1.5 U to each thyroarytenoid had a more stable dose than those who started at a dose of 2.5 U to each thyroarytenoid. Lastly, they noted the interval between injections remained constant once the optimal dose was achieved. This correlates with the findings of Brashear and colleagues,[67] who noted consistent time intervals between BoNT injections in the treatment of cervical dystonia.

6.8 Complications and Pitfalls

Treatment with BoNT results in an initial period of marked muscle weakness lasting several days, followed by a month's long plateau of somewhat milder weakening that constitutes the therapeutic effect. This is likely because of the two-stage mechanism of neural recovery from BoNT, in which partially cleaved SNAP-25 is repaired quickly in the initial phase of treatment, while completely cleaved SNAP-25 requires 3 months for full repair or replacement.[68] SNAP-25 (synaptosomal-associated protein-25) is involved in the transcytosis of the neurotransmitter acetylcholine across the cell membrane into the neuromuscular junction. The result of this initial period after thyroarytenoid injection is breathiness. Occasionally, clinically insignificant aspiration may be noted. In contrast, after PCA injection, the initial period may be marked by dyspnea. Overinjection of the PCA muscles may result in airway narrowing and a sensation of dyspnea.[69]

6.9 Conclusion

Spasmodic dysphonia is a focal laryngeal dystonia of central nervous system origin. Surgical treatment options have been either disappointing or insufficiently studied. The treatment of choice currently is BoNT injections into selected laryngeal muscles. Proper injection technique and carefully tailored dosing schedules provide patients with a safe and effective treatment.

6.10 Key Points and Pearls

- Spasmodic dysphonia is classified as a focal primary dystonia of the larynx affecting voice production. Voice patterns can be adductor (strangled voice breaks) or abductor (breathy voice breaks) predominant.
- The diagnosis of spasmodic dysphonia is clinical, based principally on perceptual analysis of the voice, complemented by the laryngoscopic examination and appropriate clinical history.
- Botulinum neurotoxin (BoNT) injection into the larynx for symptomatic control of spasmodic dysphonia has been the gold standard of treatment for most of that time, endorsed as primary therapy by the American Academy of Otolaryngology—Head and Neck Surgery.
- Laryngeal electromyography-guided injections have demonstrated safety and reliability over 30 years of treatment; however, there are various methods of injections. Effective treatments can be rendered in a variety of approaches based on the experience and skill of the injector.
- The target muscle for BoNT injection depends on the relative adductor and abductor features of the spasmodic dysphonia.
- About 12 to 15% of patients with spasmodic dysphonia have a positive family history and genetic testing shows promise as a diagnostic modality and with growing advances in brain mapping and neurogenetics, the neurological underpinnings of spasmodic dysphonia and other laryngeal dystonias are being discovered.

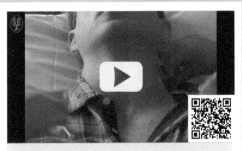

Video 6.1 Abductor spasmodic dysphonia (laryngeal dystonia). This patient has breathy breaks on connected speech segments accompanied by facial twitching. His abductor breaks require treatment of the posterior cricoarytenoid (PCA) muscle(s). First, a small amount of xylocaine is placed via the membrane into the subglottis. His injection is given via the cricothyroid membrane with a hollow-bore Teflon-coated EMG needle. The needle is placed through the membrane, through the air passage, and through the rostrum of the cricoid cartilage until the PCA muscle is impaled, whereupon a burst of electrical activity is seen on EMG. The PCA is then injected with 3.75 U/0.15 mL. Both PCA muscles are not done simultaneously, so as to avoid stridor or an airway emergency. [1:28]

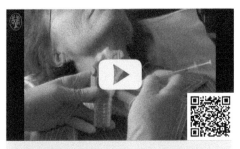

Video 6.3 Adductor spasmodic dysphonia. A hollow-bore Teflon-coated EMG needle is used via the cricothyroid membrane to inject the thyroarytenoid muscle complex. Once the muscle is engaged, the patient is asked to phonate and electrical activity is seen on the EMG: on average, 1.0 U/0.1 mL in each muscle. [1:18]

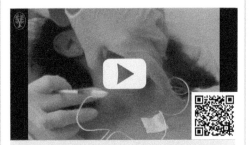

Video 6.2 Abductor spasmodic dysphonia. In these two patients, the laryngeal complex is rotated, and the EMG needle is passed posterior to the posterior lamina, through the inferior constrictor muscle, and impales the PCA muscle over the back side of the cricoid rostrum. The patients are asked to "sniff," activating the muscle, and 3.75 U/0.15 mL of Botox is injected. [2:04]

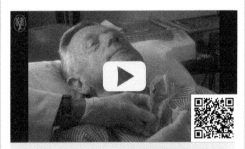

Video 6.4 Adductor spasmodic dysphonia. Another example of the transcricothyroid membrane approach to injecting the TA muscle complex with EMG guidance. An average of 1.0 U/0.1 mL is given bilaterally. [1:01]

References

[1] Traube L. Zue Lehre von den Larynxaffectionene biem Ileotyphus. Berlin: Verlag Von August Hisschwald; 1871:674–678

[2] Schnitzler J. Klinischer Atlas der Laryngologie Nebst Anleitung zur Deagnose und Therapie der Krankheiten des Kehldopfes und der Luftrohre. Vienna: Braumuller; 1895:215

[3] Gowers WR. Manual of Diseases of the Nervous System. London: Churchill; 1899

[4] Dedo HH, Behlau MS. Recurrent laryngeal nerve section for spastic dysphonia: 5- to 14-year preliminary results in the

first 300 patients. Ann Otol Rhinol Laryngol.; 100(4, Pt 1): 274–279

[5] Marsden CD, Sheehy MP. Spastic dysphonia, Meige disease, and torsion dystonia. Neurology.; 32(10):1202–1203

[6] Blitzer A, Brin MF, Fahn S, Lovelace RE. Clinical and laboratory characteristics of focal laryngeal dystonia: study of 110 cases. Laryngoscope.; 98(6, Pt 1):636–640

[7] Blitzer A, Brin MF, Simonyan K, Ozelius LJ, Frucht SJ.. Phenomenology, genetics, and CNS network abnormalities in laryngeal dystonia: a 30-year experience. Laryngoscope.; 128(Suppl 1): S1–S9

[8] Simonyan K, Berman BD, Herscovitch P, Hallett M. Abnormal striatal dopaminergic neurotransmission during rest and task production in spasmodic dysphonia. J Neurosci.; 33(37): 14705–14714

[9] Brin MF, Blitzer A, Stewart C, et al. Treatment of spasmodic dysphonia (laryngeal dystonia) with injections of Botulinum toxin: review and technical aspects. In: Blitzer A, Brin MF, Ramig LO, et al., eds. Neurological Disorders of the Larynx. New York: Thieme; 1992

[10] Hillel AD. The study of laryngeal muscle activity in normal human subjects and in patients with laryngeal dystonia using multiple fine-wire electromyography. Laryngoscope.; 111(4 Pt 2) Suppl 97:1–47

[11] Marion MH, Klap P, Perrin A, Cohen M. Stridor and focal laryngeal dystonia. Lancet.; 339(8791):457–458

[12] Chitkara A, Meyer T, Keidar A, Blitzer A. Singer's dystonia: first report of a variant of spasmodic dysphonia. Ann Otol Rhinol Laryngol.; 115(2):89–92

[13] Childs L, Rickert S, Murry T, Blitzer A, Sulica L. Patient perceptions of factors leading to spasmodic dysphonia: a combined clinical experience of 350 patients. Laryngoscope.; 121(10):2195–2198

[14] Aronson A. Abductor spastic dysphonia. In: Aronson A, ed. Clinical Voice Disorders, 2nd ed. New York: Thieme; 1985

[15] Cannito MP, Johnson JP. Spastic dysphonia: a continuum disorder. J Commun Disord.; 14(3):215–233

[16] Davis PJ, Boone DR, Carroll RL, Darveniza P, Harrison GA. Adductor spastic dysphonia: heterogeneity of physiologic and phonatory characteristics. Ann Otol Rhinol Laryngol.; 97 (2, Pt 1):179–185

[17] Blitzer A, Lovelace RE, Brin MF, Fahn S, Fink ME. Electromyographic findings in focal laryngeal dystonia (spastic dysphonia). Ann Otol Rhinol Laryngol.; 94(6, Pt 1):591–594

[18] Leonard R, Kendall K. Differentiation of spasmodic and psychogenic dysphonias with phonoscopic evaluation. Laryngoscope.; 109(2, Pt 1):295–300

[19] Ludlow CL, Domangue R, Sharma D, et al. Consensus-based attributes for identifying patients with spasmodic dysphonia and other voice disorders. JAMA Otolaryngol Head Neck Surg.; 144(8):657–665

[20] Ludlow CL, Adler CH, Berke GS, et al. Research priorities in spasmodic dysphonia. Otolaryngol Head Neck Surg.; 139(4): 495–505

[21] Zwirner P, Murry T, Swenson M, Woodson GE. Acoustic changes in spasmodic dysphonia after botulinum toxin injection. J Voice.; 5:78–84

[22] Sapienza CM, Walton S, Murry T. Adductor spasmodic dysphonia and muscular tension dysphonia: acoustic analysis of sustained phonation and reading. J Voice.; 14(4):502–520

[23] Koufman JA. A classification of laryngeal dystonias. The Visible Voice.; 1:1–5

[24] Schaefer SD, Freeman FJ, Watson BC, et al. Vocal tract electromyographic abnormalities in spasmodic dysphonia: a preliminary report. Trans Am Laryngol Assoc.; 108:187

[25] Watson BC, Schaefer SD, Freeman FJ, Dembowski J, Kondraske G, Roark R. Laryngeal electromyographic activity in adductor and abductor spasmodic dysphonia. J Speech Hear Res.; 34 (3):473–482

[26] Nash EA, Ludlow CL. Laryngeal muscle activity during speech breaks in adductor spasmodic dysphonia. Laryngoscope.; 106 (4):484–489

[27] Sataloff RT, Mandel S, Mann EA, Ludlow CL. Practice parameter: laryngeal electromyography (an evidence-based review). Otolaryngol Head Neck Surg.; 130(6):770–779

[28] de Gusmão CM, Fuchs T, Moses A, et al. Dystonia-causing mutations as a contribution to the etiology of spasmodic dysphonia. Otolaryngol Head Neck Surg.; 155(4):624–628

[29] Mor N, Simonyan K, Blitzer A. Central voice production and pathophysiology of spasmodic dysphonia. Laryngoscope.; 128(1):177–183

[30] Blitzer A, Brin MF, Stewart CF. Botulinum toxin management of spasmodic dysphonia (laryngeal dystonia): a 12-year experience in more than 900 patients. Laryngoscope.; 125(8): 1751–1757

[31] Boutsen F, Cannito MP, Taylor M, Bender B. Botox treatment in adductor spasmodic dysphonia: a meta-analysis. J Speech Lang Hear Res.; 45(3):469–481

[32] Whurr R, Nye C, Lorch M. Meta-analysis of botulinum toxin treatment of spasmodic dysphonia: a review of 22 studies. Int J Lang Commun Disord.; 33 Suppl:327–329

[33] Troung DD, Rontal M, Rolnick M, Aronson AE, Mistura K. Double-blind controlled study of botulinum toxin in adductor spasmodic dysphonia. Laryngoscope.; 101(6, Pt 1):630–634

[34] Byrnes ML, Thickbroom GW, Wilson SA, et al. The corticomotor representation of upper limb muscles in writer's cramp and changes following botulinum toxin injection. Brain.; 121 (Pt 5):977–988

[35] Bielamowicz S, Ludlow CL. Effects of botulinum toxin on pathophysiology in spasmodic dysphonia. Ann Otol Rhinol Laryngol.; 109(2):194–203

[36] Antonucci F, Rossi C, Gianfranceschi L, Rossetto O, Caleo M. Long-distance retrograde effects of botulinum neurotoxin A. J Neurosci.; 28(14):3689–3696

[37] Adams SG, Hunt EJ, Charles DA, Lang AE. Unilateral versus bilateral botulinum toxin injections in spasmodic dysphonia: acoustic and perceptual results. J Otolaryngol.; 22(3):171–175

[38] Adams SG, Hunt EJ, Irish JC, et al. Comparison of botulinum toxin injection procedures in adductor spasmodic dysphonia. J Otolaryngol.; 24(6):345–351

[39] Upile T, Elmiyeh B, Jerjes W, et al. Unilateral versus bilateral thyroarytenoid Botulinum toxin injections in adductor spasmodic dysphonia: a prospective study. Head Face Med.; 5:20

[40] Ford CN, Bless DM, Lowery JD. Indirect laryngoscopic approach for injection of botulinum toxin in spasmodic dysphonia. Otolaryngol Head Neck Surg.; 103(5, Pt 1):752–758

[41] Hussain A, Thiel G, Shakeel M. Trans-nasal injection of botulinum toxin. J Laryngol Otol.; 123(7):783–785

[42] Green DC, Berke GS, Ward PH, Gerratt BR. Point-touch technique of botulinum toxin injection for the treatment of spasmodic dysphonia. Ann Otol Rhinol Laryngol.; 101(11): 883–887

[43] Rhew K, Fiedler DA, Ludlow CL. Technique for injection of botulinum toxin through the flexible nasolaryngoscope. Otolaryngol Head Neck Surg.; 111(6):787–794

[44] Blitzer A, Brin MF, Fahn S. Botulinum toxin therapy for recurrent laryngeal nerve section failure for adductor laryngeal dystonia. Trans Am Laryngol Assoc.; 110:206

[45] Sulica L, Blitzer A, Brin MF, Stewart CF. Botulinum toxin management of adductor spasmodic dysphonia after failed

recurrent laryngeal nerve section. Ann Otol Rhinol Laryngol.; 112(6):499–505

[46] Ludlow CL, Naunton RF, Fujita M, Sedory SE. Spasmodic dysphonia: botulinum toxin injection after recurrent nerve surgery. Otolaryngol Head Neck Surg.; 102(2):122–131

[47] Blitzer A, Brin MF, Stewart C, Aviv JE, Fahn S. Abductor laryngeal dystonia: a series treated with botulinum toxin. Laryngoscope.; 102(2):163–167

[48] Stong BC, DelGaudio JM, Hapner ER, Johns MM, III. Safety of simultaneous bilateral botulinum toxin injections for abductor spasmodic dysphonia. Arch Otolaryngol Head Neck Surg.; 131(9):793–795

[49] Hillel AD, Maronian NC, Waugh PF, Robinson L, Klotz DA. Treatment of the interarytenoid muscle with botulinum toxin for laryngeal dystonia. Ann Otol Rhinol Laryngol.; 113(5):341–348

[50] Rumbach AF, Blitzer A, Frucht SJ, Simonyan K. An open-label study of sodium oxybate in Spasmodic dysphonia. Laryngoscope.; 127(6):1402–1407

[51] Aronson AE, De Santo LW. Adductor spastic dysphonia: three years after recurrent laryngeal nerve resection. Laryngoscope.; 93(1):1–8

[52] Netterville JL, Stone RE, Rainey C, Zealear DL, Ossoff RH. Recurrent laryngeal nerve avulsion for treatment of spastic dysphonia. Ann Otol Rhinol Laryngol.; 100(1):10–14

[53] Tucker HM. Laryngeal framework surgery in the management of spasmodic dysphonia. Preliminary report. Ann Otol Rhinol Laryngol.; 98(1, Pt 1):52–54

[54] Genack SH, Woo P, Colton RH, Goyette D. Partial thyroarytenoid myectomy: an animal study investigating a proposed new treatment for adductor spasmodic dysphonia. Otolaryngol Head Neck Surg.; 108(3):256–264

[55] Friedman M, Toriumi DM, Grybauskas VT, Applebaum EL. Implantation of a recurrent laryngeal nerve stimulator for the treatment of spastic dysphonia. Ann Otol Rhinol Laryngol.; 98(2):130–134

[56] Berke GS, Blackwell KE, Gerratt BR, Verneil A, Jackson KS, Sercarz JA. Selective laryngeal adductor denervation-reinnervation: a new surgical treatment for adductor spasmodic dysphonia. Ann Otol Rhinol Laryngol.; 108(3):227–231

[57] van Esch BF, Wegner I, Stegeman I, Grolman W. Effect of botulinum toxin and surgery among spasmodic dysphonia patients. Otolaryngol Head Neck Surg.; 156(2):238–254

[58] Mendelsohn AH, Berke GS. Surgery or botulinum toxin for adductor spasmodic dysphonia: a comparative study. Ann Otol Rhinol Laryngol.; 121(4):231–238

[59] Chang CY, Chabot P, Thomas JP. Relationship of botulinum dosage to duration of side effects and normal voice in adductor spasmodic dysphonia. Otolaryngol Head Neck Surg.; 136(6):894–899

[60] Adler CH, Bansberg SF, Krein-Jones K, Hentz JG. Safety and efficacy of botulinum toxin type B (Myobloc) in adductor spasmodic dysphonia. Mov Disord.; 19(9):1075–1079

[61] Blitzer A. Botulinum toxin A and B: a comparative dosing study for spasmodic dysphonia. Otolaryngol Head Neck Surg.; 133(6):836–838

[62] Klotz DA, Maronian NC, Waugh PF, Shahinfar A, Robinson L, Hillel AD. Findings of multiple muscle involvement in a study of 214 patients with laryngeal dystonia using fine-wire electromyography. Ann Otol Rhinol Laryngol.; 113(8):602–612

[63] Cooper MH. Anatomy of the larynx. In: Blitzer A, Brin MF, Ramig LO, eds. Neurologic Disorders of the Larynx. New York: Thieme; 2009:198–199

[64] Meleca RJ, Hogikyan ND, Bastian RW. A comparison of methods of botulinum toxin injection for abductory spasmodic dysphonia. Otolaryngol Head Neck Surg.; 117(5):487–492

[65] Ludlow CL, Naunton RF, Terada S, Anderson BJ. Successful treatment of selected cases of abductor spasmodic dysphonia using botulinum toxin injection. Otolaryngol Head Neck Surg.; 104(6):849–855

[66] Holden PK, Vokes DE, Taylor MB, Till JA, Crumley RL. Long-term botulinum toxin dose consistency for treatment of adductor spasmodic dysphonia. Ann Otol Rhinol Laryngol.; 116(12):891–896

[67] Brashear A, Hogan P, Wooten-Watts M, Marchetti A, Magar R, Martin J. Longitudinal assessment of the dose consistency of botulinum toxin type A (BOTOX) for cervical dystonia. Adv Ther.; 22(1):49–55

[68] de Paiva A, Meunier FA, Molgó J, Aoki KR, Dolly JO. Functional repair of motor endplates after botulinum neurotoxin type A poisoning: biphasic switch of synaptic activity between nerve sprouts and their parent terminals. Proc Natl Acad Sci U S A.; 96(6):3200–3205

[69] Klein AM, Stong BC, Wise J, DelGaudio JM, Hapner ER, Johns MM, III. Vocal outcome measures after bilateral posterior cricoarytenoid muscle botulinum toxin injections for abductor spasmodic dysphonia. Otolaryngol Head Neck Surg.; 139(3):421–423

7

Botulinum Neurotoxin for Cervical Dystonia

Tanya K. Meyer, Joel Guss, and Ronda E. Alexander

Summary

Cervical dystonia (CD) is the most common focal dystonia and causes significant functional deficits. The pathophysiology is poorly understood, although there is a genetic component in some individuals. The efficacy of oral medications is limited. The mainstay of treatment is the injection of botulinum neurotoxin into the affected cervical musculature. Deep brain stimulation has been shown to have success for certain cases of dystonia and tremor. This chapter discusses the appropriate workup required and the injection technique for CD.

Keywords: botulinum neurotoxin, cervical dystonia, focal dystonia, torticollis

7.1 Introduction

Cervical dystonia or CD is the most common focal dystonia.[1] It results in the sustained contraction of the cervical musculature, leading to abnormal posturing of the neck, head, and shoulder. The injection of botulinum neurotoxin (BoNT) into the overactive muscles of CD patients can effectively treat the abnormal neck movements and pain caused by this disorder. The abnormal movements of the neck and head can result in twisting (torticollis), tilting (laterocollis), flexion (anterocollis), or extension (retro-collis). Additional movements are shoulder elevation and lateral movement of the head/neck with relation to the chest wall.

7.2 Epidemiology

The incidence of CD is 9 to 30 per 100,000 people in the United States, and the prevalence may vary among ethnic groups.[1,2] Studies have shown a higher incidence among women, with an approximate 2:1 female-to-male ratio.[3] In greater than 70% of cases, the disease begins between the fourth and sixth decades of life, with a peak incidence in the fifth decade.[4] A family history of dystonia is seen in 12%. Progression of dystonia to other anatomic areas is seen in up to one-third of cases.[3]

Symptoms typically worsen over the course of the first 5 years before stabilizing. Spontaneous remission is seen in 10 to 20% of individuals lasting days to years, although these are temporary and most patients eventually relapse.[3,5] Employment status is significantly affected by CD, with over 30% requiring reduced work hours or reduced responsibilities and 19% resulting in loss of employment.[6]

7.3 Pathophysiology

As in all dystonia, the pathophysiology of idiopathic CD is not well understood, although it is generally thought to be an abnormality in central motor processing.

There is a genetic component to the development of dystonia, but trauma and drug exposure can also be a precedent to focal dystonia.[7] The use of neuroleptics or metoclopramide can be associated with acute onset of dystonia or tardive dystonia, which can be accompanied by other more typical tardive movements such as orofacial dyskinesia and akathisia.[8] Currently, the main theories are decreased central inhibition, sensory deficit with sensorimotor mismatch, aberrant neuroplasticity, and abnormal basal ganglia discharge.[9,10,11,12,13,14] Although any muscle in the neck may be involved, ▶ Table 7.1 lists the common muscles with the associated head/neck movements. There may be multiple muscles involved with co-contraction of agonist and antagonist muscles.

7.4 Clinical Manifestation

Idiopathic CD usually begins with abnormal head/neck movements before progressing to other areas. Head tremor and neck spasms are cardinal features of CD, and the majority of affected patients complain of pain. Approximately half of patients are able to identify a sensory trick, or *geste antagoniste*, to help control their abnormal neck spasms.[15] Typically, this trick constitutes placing the hand on the side of the face or neck, and this contact reduces the muscle spasm without actually mechanically opposing the spasm. Some patients can even imagine the sensory trick to diminish symptomatic spasms.[16] The pathophysiology of the sensory trick is unknown. Although early in the course of disease these tricks are helpful in most patients, they tend to lose effectiveness as the disease progresses.

Additional palliative factors include relaxation, alcoholic beverages, and "morning benefit," in which symptoms are less intense just after waking. CD is exacerbated by activity, stress, and fatigue.

Table 7.1 Typical muscles involved in cervical dystonia

Movement	Muscles involved
Rotational: torticollis	Ipsilateral semispinalis cervicis
	Ipsilateral levator scapulae
	Ipsilateral splenius cervicis
Rotational: torticaput	Ipsilateral splenius capitis
	Ipsilateral obliquus capitis inferior
	Contralateral sternocleidomastoid
	Contralateral trapezius
	Contralateral semispinalis capitis
Laterocollis	Ipsilateral sternocleidomastoid
	Ipsilateral splenius capitis
	Ipsilateral scalene complex
	Ipsilateral levator scapulae
	Ipsilateral trapezius
Shoulder elevation	Ipsilateral levator scapulae
	Ipsilateral trapezius
Retrocollis	Bilateral splenius capitis[a]
	Bilateral semispinalis capitis[a]
	Bilateral upper trapezius[a]
Anterocollis	Bilateral sternocleidomastoid[a]
	Bilateral scalene complex[a]
	Bilateral submental complex[a]

Source: Data from Brashear A. The botulinum toxins in the treatment of cervical dystonia. Semin Neurol 2001;21(1):85–90; and from Walker FO. Botulinum toxin therapy for cervical dystonia. Phys Med Rehabil Clin N Am 2003;14:749–766; and from Jost WH, Tatu L. Selection of muscles for botulinum toxin injections in cervical dystonia. Mov Disord Clin Pract 2015;2:224–226.

[a]For bilateral injections, decrease the individual dose by 50 to 60% to avoid unwanted dysphagia in the anterior injections or neck weakness and difficulty holding the head straight in the posterior injections.

On physical examination, muscles should be palpated for hypertrophy, activity, and contracture/fibrosis, although it may be difficult to differentiate these conditions. Areas of pain should be noted. By convention, the direction of the rotation is defined by the chin, so right-turning torticollis means that the chin deviates to the patient's right. Abnormal head and neck postures can occur in multiple planes. Rotational torticollis occurs around the longitudinal axis, laterocollis rotates the head in the coronal plane tilting the ear to the shoulder, and anterocollis and retrocollis rotate the head in the sagittal plane. In addition, there may be sagittal or lateral deviation of the base of the neck from the midline. Deviations in only one plane are seen in less than one-third of patients.[5]

It is important to remember that an abnormal head and neck posture with cervical musculature spasm can be a manifestation of other disease processes, both acute and chronic. Thus, a full history and diagnostic workup should be performed. Wilson disease should be excluded in all patients younger than 50 years through evaluation of serum ceruloplasmin and slit lamp examination. Lesions and abnormalities of the brain, posterior fossa, and spinal cord can be excluded through imaging studies. A full neurologic examination should be performed. The presence of fasciculations, cerebellar signs, cranial nerve weakness, or cortical dysfunction should alert the clinician that there may be additional pathology present. The differential diagnoses of torticollis are as follows:

- Cervical spine fracture or disease.
- Peritonsillar or retropharyngeal abscess.
- Drug reaction (tardive dystonia).
  - Neuroleptics: droperidol, haloperidol, pimozide, Thorazine, Compazine.
  - Dopamine receptor antagonists: metoclopramide.
- Wilson disease.
- Klippel-Feil syndrome.
- Sandifer syndrome.
- Bobble-head doll syndrome (with third ventricle cyst).
- Progressive supranuclear palsy.
- Posterior fossa tumor.
- Spinal cord tumor or syrinx.
- Multiple sclerosis.

- Systemic lupus erythematosus.
- Huntington disease.
- Psychogenic dystonia.

7.5 Management

7.5.1 Medical Therapy

Although the efficacy of oral drug therapy is limited, there are medications that can ameliorate the severity of CD, or serve as adjuncts in the treatment of CD (► Table 7.2). Anticholinergic medications such as trihexyphenidyl or benztropine have been shown to have some effect in about a third of patients, but may be poorly tolerated due to anticholinergic side effects of dry mouth, constipation, confusion, and blurred vision. Benzodiazepines, particularly clonazepam, may also show some effect.[17]

7.5.2 Surgery

Denervation and myotomy techniques to address the abnormally functioning musculature have been explored for centuries. Isaac Minnius sectioned the sternocleidomastoid muscle to address CD in 1641. Campbell de Morgan in London sectioned the spinal accessory nerve in 1866. William Halsted, Harvey Cushing, John Finney, Theodor Kocher, Fritz De Quervain, and Guillaume Depuytren are among the reported names of esteemed surgeons who have attempted surgical amelioration of torticollis.[23] Although cervical rhizotomy was the standard technique prior to the introduction of BoNT therapy, it has been largely abandoned due to limited efficacy in the face of a relatively high burden of side effects. In general, it is thought that surgical denervation is an option for patients refractory to BoNT injections.[24,25]

Table 7.2 Medications used for dystonia

Names	Mechanism	Beneficial effects	Adverse effects
Trihexyphenidyl Ethopropazine Benztropine	Anticholinergic	In a double-blind placebo-controlled trial using trihexyphenidyl, 71% had a clinically significant response, with 42% maintaining long-term benefit[18] In a prospective, randomized, double-blind controlled trial, botulinum neurotoxin type A (BoNT-A) was shown to be more effective in treatment of abnormal movements and pain as compared with trihexyphenidyl[19] Anticholinergics are considered the most beneficial oral pharmacologic agent[20]	Dry mouth, blurred vision, imbalance, forgetfulness, fatigue, depression, micturition disturbance Can use pyridostigmine to overcome peripheral effects[21] Can use pilocarpine eyedrops for blurred vision[21] Dose usually limited by side effects Need to discontinue slowly to prevent rare occurrence of neuroleptic malignant syndrome
Benzodiazepines	GABA agonist	Muscle relaxation, works at spinal cord level A review of over 500 patients treated over 15 y showed marked improvement in 63% of patients with idiopathic dystonia[22]	Sedation
Baclofen	GABA-B agonist		Sedation
Tetrabenazine	Presynaptic catecholamine depleting agent		Akathisia, depression, sedation, fatigue, insomnia, anxiety, Parkinsonism

Brain lesioning has been used since the early 1940s for the treatment of CD, with variable results. Targets include selected regions of the basal ganglia and thalamus. These procedures can cause significant side effects including weakness, dysphagia, and dysarthria in 6 to 47% of patients.[26] These destructive techniques have been supplanted by deep brain stimulation (DBS) due to the more favorable risk profile and promising results.[27]

Deep brain stimulation is used to treat several types of movement disorders (chronic pain, Parkinson, depression, dystonia, tremor, Tourette syndrome) and has the advantage over brain lesioning of being reversible and adjustable. There are reported neuropsychiatric side effects, including mood disorders and hypersexual behavior, but these can theoretically be modulated by adjustment of the stimulation.[28] Permanent cognitive complications are rare. Studies have shown excellent therapeutic efficacy and safety for DBS in patients with disabling CD.[27,29]

7.5.3 Chemodenervation

The introduction of chemodenervation with BoNT of the cervical musculature has dramatically improved the prognosis and quality of life of patients with CD. Off-label treatment of patients with CD with BoNT-A started in the late 1980s and, due to an excellent effect, was quickly accepted and widely used. Since 2000, the use of BoNT-A and BoNT-B (onabotulinumtoxinA and rimabotulinumtoxinB) has been a Food and Drug Administration (FDA)-approved indication for CD and has become the favored treatment for this condition. In 2009 abobotulinumtoxinA and in 2010 incobotulinumtoxinA were FDA approved for CD.[17]

Botulinum neurotoxin can cause weakness of the injected muscles, leading to atrophy and ameliorating the spasmodic contractions. The injections can alleviate the abnormal head postures, tremor and pain for approximately 3 to 4 months. This therapy has been proved effective in many double-blind placebo-controlled and open trails with fewer side effects than other pharmacologic therapies or surgical procedures prior to the advent of DBS.[30,31]

All the commonly commercially available BoNT brands have shown efficacy compared to placebo in treating CD.[32] There are dosing differences between the different serotypes of BoNT and also different brands of the same serotype. Although a set of conversion formula has not been established, studies have recommended approximate ratios as listed in ▶ Table 7.3.[30,31,33,34,35] Although there is variability in the number of muscles injected, the number of injections per muscle, and the dose of BoNT used, the average dose for CD is 200 U of onabotulinumtoxinA or 500 U of abobotulinumtoxinA.[30]

Direct efficacy comparisons among brands and serotypes have been reported. A Cochrane review of studies comparing onabotulinumtoxinA and rimabotulinumtoxinB evaluated efficacy and adverse events concluding that overall efficacy was similar, although treatment with rimabotulinumtoxinB confers an increased risk of sore throat and dry mouth as an adverse event.[42] One of the included studies also showed that the duration of benefit from rimabotulinumtoxinB was approximately 2 weeks shorter than with onabotulinumtoxinA.[40] IncobotulinumtoxinA has been shown similar clinical efficacy to onabotulinumtoxinA with a similar side-effect profile.[35]

Overall, approximately one-third of patients treated at least once choose not to continue chronic injections because of an unsatisfactory response, the lack of effect, or the high cost of treatment.[43,44] Additionally, 15 to 30% of patients are cited as primary nonresponders (never benefit from injections); the nonresponse is thought to be due to muscle contractures, inadequate dosing, inaccurate muscle selection, or inaccessible dystonic musculature. Anterocollis is particularly nonresponsive to injections because of involvement of the inaccessible deep anterior prevertebral musculature. Secondary treatment failures (loss of efficacy following previous successful injections) are thought to occur in 10 to 15% of patients, and up to one-third of patients are found to have antibodies to BoNT by the mouse neutralization assay.[15,45] IncobotulinumtoxinA is a highly purified formulation of BoNT-A that is free of other complex proteins and has shown promise in having a reduced incidence of neutralizing antibody formation to date.[46]

Table 7.3 Dose conversion between neurotoxin types/brands

BoNT type	Name	Brand name	Dose conversion to ona-BoNT-A	References
BoNT-A	OnabotulinumtoxinA	Botox	1:1	–
BoNT-A	AbobotulinumtoxinA	Dysport	1:3–4	Sampaio et al (1997)[36] Bentivoglio et al (2012)[37]
BoNT-A	IncobotulinumtoxinA	Xeomin	1:1	Benecke et al (2005)[38] Roggenkämper et al (2006)[39]
BoNT-B	RimabotulinumtoxinB	Myobloc/Neurobloc	1:40–60	Comella et al (2005)[40] Pappert et al (2008)[41]

7.6 Injection Technique

Successful treatment of patients depends on knowledge of neck anatomy and accurate assessment of involved musculature. The sternocleidomastoid, trapezius, splenius capitis, and levator scapulae are most commonly injected (▶ Fig. 7.1; ▶ Fig. 7.2; ▶ Fig. 7.3; ▶ Fig. 7.4; ▶ Fig. 7.5; ▶ Fig. 7.6).[47,48]

Although selection of injection sites using clinical exam and needle place-ment using anatomic landmarks are efficacious,[8,49] Comella et al[50] reported a significantly greater magnitude of improvement in patients whose injections were administered under electromyographic guidance compared to those in whom only anatomic localization and clinical examination was used. Ultrasound guidance is an additional useful technique for deep posterior muscular injections or in individuals with distorted anatomy.[51]

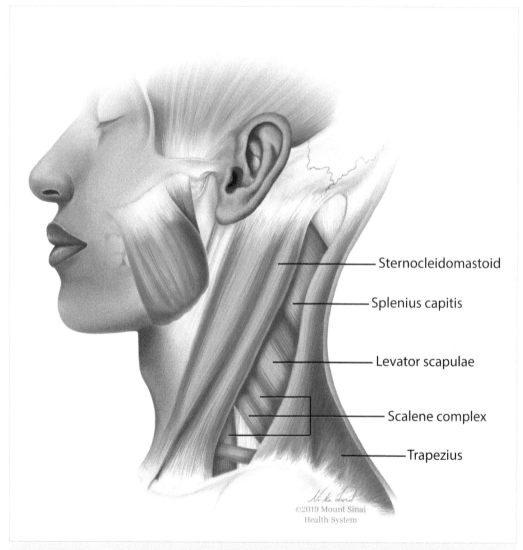

Sternocleidomastoid

Splenius capitis

Levator scapulae

Scalene complex

Trapezius

©2019 Mount Sinai
Health System

Fig. 7.1 Lateral view of neck muscles typically injected for cervical dystonia. (Printed with permission from Mount Sinai Health System.)

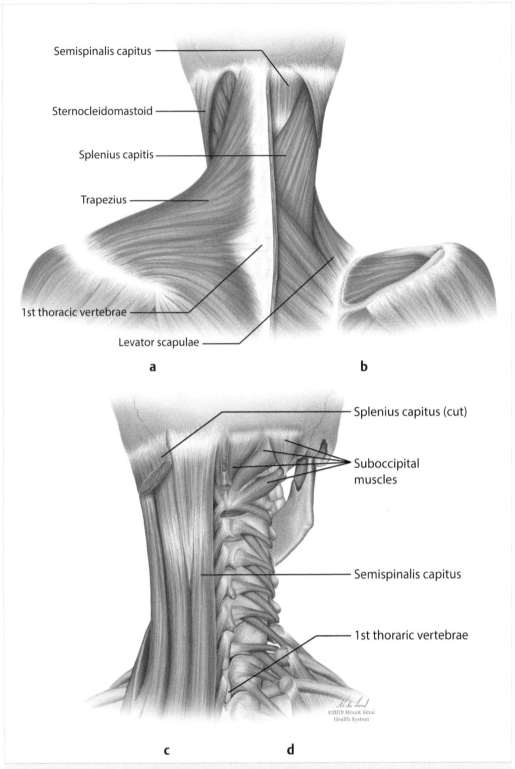

Fig. 7.2 (a) Posterior view of neck muscles. (b) Right trapezius muscle removed. (c) Left trapezius and splenius capitis removed. (d) Right trapezius, splenius capitis and semispinalis capitis removed showing the suboccipital muscles. (Printed with permission from Mount Sinai Health System.)

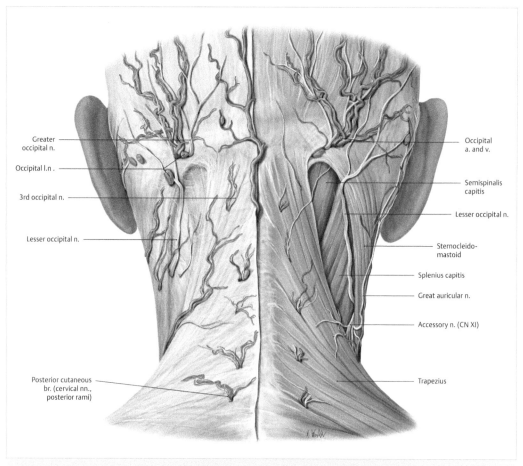

Fig. 7.3 Splenius capitis muscle. (From Gilroy AM et al. Atlas of Anatomy. 1st Ed. New York: Thieme Medical Publishers; 2008. Based on: Schuenke M, Schulte E, Schumacher U. THIEME Atlas of Anatomy: Head and Neuroanatomy. Illustrations by Voll M and Wesker K. 1st Ed. New York: Thieme Medical Publishers; 2008.)

Rotational head turning is the simplest symptom to treat and usually involves injection of the contralateral sternocleidomastoid and the ipsilateral splenius capitis and semispinalis capitis. For refractory cases, deeper cervical musculature may need treatment including the ipsilateral obliquus capitis inferior.[48] These patients may also have pain, which may give some indication as to the appropriate location of the injection.[52] It is important to use the lowest dose possible and to maximize the time between injections, to minimize side effects, and also to minimize antigenic load. For the sternocleidomastoid, the injections are given in the rostral third of the muscle, which helps limit dysphagia. Injections of the posterior neck musculature can cause some neck weakness (such as lifting the chin off of the chest) and rarely difficulty opening the jaw if the injections track anteriorly toward the pterygoid musculature. Ipsilateral laterocollis (head tilt) is usually caused by involvement of the ipsilateral splenius capitis, levator scapulae, and sternocleidomastoid. Injections of the levator scapulae have rarely been associated with brachial plexus injury or pneumothorax.[53] Retrocollis and head tremor can be treated with splenius capitis and semi-

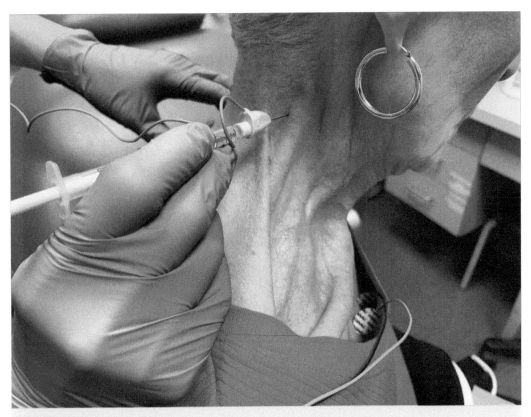

Fig. 7.4 Semispinalis capitis injection.

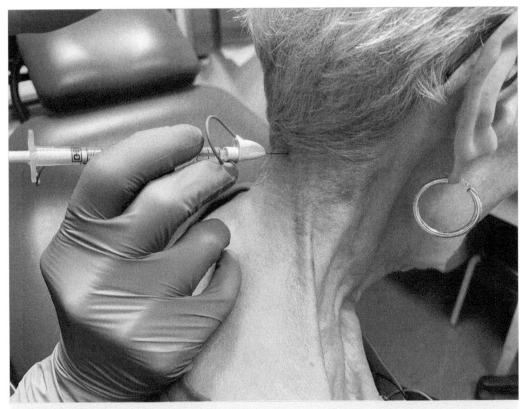

Fig. 7.5 Levator scapulae injection.

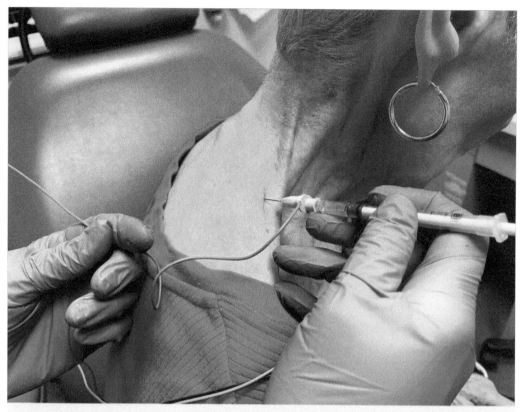

Fig. 7.6 Trapezius muscle injection.

spinalis capitis injections. Anterocollis is the most difficult movement to treat and involves injection of the scalene complex and of the anterior deep paravertebral musculature, which is difficult to access transcutaneously.

7.7 Conclusion

Cervical dystonia is the most common form of focal dystonia and affects more than 90,000 people in the United States. It is important to perform a full neurologic evaluation to exclude other causes of abnormal neck movement in new cases. CD causes significant patient disability and loss of quality of life. BoNT chemodenervation is the most common treatment for

these patients and can alleviate the abnormal neck postures, relieve pain, and prevent the muscle fibrosis and cervical spine degenerative complications associated with the constant abnormal muscle spasms.[54]

7.8 Key Points/Pearls

- Botulinum neurotoxin can be used to successfully and safely treat cervical dystonia.
- Deep brain stimulation may be a surgical option for selected patients.
- It is important to use the lowest dose possible and to maximize the time between injections, to minimize side effects and also minimize antigenic load.

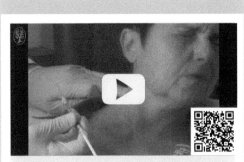

Video 7.1 Cervical dystonia (torticollis). This patient has laterocollis with a head tilt and rotation to the right. She receives EMG-guided injections of 5 U/0.1 mL in multiple sites of the following muscles: sternocleidomastoid, splenius capitis, platysma, trapezius, and occipitalis. [6:52]

References

[1] Nutt JG, Muenter MD, Melton LJ, III, Aronson A, Kurland LT. Epidemiology of dystonia in Rochester, Minnesota. Adv Neurol.; 50:361–365

[2] Claypool DW, Duane DD, Ilstrup DM, Melton LJ, III. Epidemiology and outcome of cervical dystonia (spasmodic torticollis) in Rochester, Minnesota. Mov Disord.; 10(5):608–614

[3] Jahanshahi M, Marion MH, Marsden CD. Natural history of adult-onset idiopathic torticollis. Arch Neurol.; 47(5): 548–552

[4] Duane DD. Spasmodic torticollis. Adv Neurol.; 49:135–150

[5] Chan J, Brin MF, Fahn S. Idiopathic cervical dystonia: clinical characteristics. Mov Disord.; 6(2):119–126

[6] Molho ES, Agarwal N, Regan K, Higgins DS, Factor SA. Effect of cervical dystonia on employment: a retrospective analysis of the ability of treatment to restore premorbid employment status. Mov Disord.; 24(9):1384–1387

[7] Tarsy D. Comparison of acute- and delayed-onset posttraumatic cervical dystonia. Mov Disord.; 13(3):481–485

[8] Walker FO. Botulinum toxin therapy for cervical dystonia. Phys Med Rehabil Clin N Am.; 14(4):749–766, vi

[9] Hallett M. Dystonia: abnormal movements result from loss of inhibition. Adv Neurol.; 94:1–9

[10] Molloy FM, Carr TD, Zeuner KE, Dambrosia JM, Hallett M. Abnormalities of spatial discrimination in focal and generalized dystonia. Brain.; 126(Pt 10):2175–2182

[11] Sanger TD, Merzenich MM. Computational model of the role of sensory disorganization in focal task-specific dystonia. J Neurophysiol.; 84(5):2458–2464

[12] Thickbroom GW, Byrnes ML, Stell R, Mastaglia FL. Reversible reorganisation of the motor cortical representation of the hand in cervical dystonia. Mov Disord.; 18(4):395–402

[13] Vitek JL, Chockkan V, Zhang JY, et al. Neuronal activity in the basal ganglia in patients with generalized dystonia and hemiballismus. Ann Neurol.; 46(1):22–35

[14] Zhuang P, Li Y, Hallett M. Neuronal activity in the basal ganglia and thalamus in patients with dystonia. Clin Neurophysiol.; 115(11):2542–2557

[15] Jankovic J, Leder S, Warner D, Schwartz K. Cervical dystonia: clinical findings and associated movement disorders. Neurology.; 41(7):1088–1091

[16] Müller J, Wissel J, Masuhr F, Ebersbach G, Wenning GK, Poewe W. Clinical characteristics of the geste antagoniste in cervical dystonia. J Neurol.; 248(6):478–482

[17] Jankovic J. Medical treatment of dystonia. Mov Disord.; 28(7): 1001–1012

[18] Burke RE, Fahn S, Marsden CD. Torsion dystonia: a double-blind, prospective trial of high-dosage trihexyphenidyl. Neurology.; 36(2):160–164

[19] Brans JW, Lindeboom R, Snoek JW, et al. Botulinum toxin versus trihexyphenidyl in cervical dystonia: a prospective, randomized, double-blind controlled trial. Neurology.; 46(4): 1066–1072

[20] Greene P, Shale H, Fahn S. Analysis of open-label trials in torsion dystonia using high dosages of anticholinergics and other drugs. Mov Disord.; 3(1):46–60

[21] Fahn S. Systemic therapy of dystonia. Can J Neurol Sci.; 14(3) Suppl:528–532

[22] Jankovic J, Beach J. Long-term effects of tetrabenazine in hyperkinetic movement disorders. Neurology.; 48(2):358–362

[23] Vogel TD, Pendleton C, Quiñones-Hinojosa A, Cohen-Gadol AA. Surgery for cervical dystonia: the emergence of denervation and myotomy techniques and the contributions of early surgeons at The Johns Hopkins Hospital. J Neurosurg Spine.; 12(3):280–285

[24] Cohen-Gadol AA, Ahlskog JE, Matsumoto JY, Swenson MA, McClelland RL, Davis DH. Selective peripheral denervation for the treatment of intractable spasmodic torticollis: experience with 168 patients at the Mayo Clinic. J Neurosurg.; 98 (6):1247–1254

[25] Ford B, Louis ED, Greene P, Fahn S. Outcome of selective ramisectomy for botulinum toxin resistant torticollis. J Neurol Neurosurg Psychiatry.; 65(4):472–478

[26] Yoshor D, Hamilton WJ, Ondo W, Jankovic J, Grossman RG. Comparison of thalamotomy and pallidotomy for the treatment of dystonia. Neurosurgery.; 48(4):818–824, discussion 824–826

[27] Krauss JK. Surgical treatment of dystonia. Eur J Neurol.; 17 Suppl 1:97–101

[28] Burn DJ, Tröster AI. Neuropsychiatric complications of medical and surgical therapies for Parkinson's disease. J Geriatr Psychiatry Neurol.; 17(3):172–180

[29] Ostrem JL, San Luciano M, Dodenhoff KA, et al. Subthalamic nucleus deep brain stimulation in isolated dystonia: a 3-year follow-up study. Neurology.; 88(1):25–35

[30] Jankovic J. Treatment of cervical dystonia with botulinum toxin. Mov Disord.; 19 Suppl 8:S109–S115

[31] Marchetti A, Magar R, Findley L, et al. Retrospective evaluation of the dose of Dysport and BOTOX in the management of cervical dystonia and blepharospasm: the REAL DOSE study. Mov Disord.; 20(8):937–944

[32] Han Y, Stevens AL, Dashtipour K, Hauser RA, Mari Z. A mixed treatment comparison to compare the efficacy and safety of botulinum toxin treatments for cervical dystonia. J Neurol.; 263(4):772–780

[33] Dressler D. Botulinum toxin for treatment of dystonia. Eur J Neurol.; 17 Suppl 1:88–96

[34] Ranoux D, Gury C, Fondarai J, Mas JL, Zuber M. Respective potencies of Botox and Dysport: a double blind, randomised, crossover study in cervical dystonia. J Neurol Neurosurg Psychiatry.; 72(4):459–462

[35] Benecke R. Xeomin in the treatment of cervical dystonia. Eur J Neurol.; 16 Suppl 2:6–10

[36] Sampaio C, Ferreira JJ, Simões F, et al. DYSBOT: a single-blind, randomized parallel study to determine whether any differences can be detected in the efficacy and tolerability of two formulations of botulinum toxin type A–Dysport and Botox–assuming a ratio of 4:1. Mov Disord.; 12(6):1013–1018

[37] Bentivoglio AR, Ialongo T, Bove F, De Nigris F, Fasano A. Retrospective evaluation of the dose equivalence of Botox(®) and Dysport (®) in the management of blepharospasm and hemifacial spasm: a novel paradigm for a never ending story. Neurol Sci.; 33(2):261–267

[38] Benecke R, Jost WH, Kanovsky P, Ruzicka E, Comes G, Grafe S. A new botulinum toxin type A free of complexing proteins for treatment of cervical dystonia. Neurology.; 64(11):1949–1951

[39] Roggenkämper P, Jost WH, Bihari K, Comes G, Grafe S, NT 201 Blepharospasm Study Team. Efficacy and safety of a new Botulinum Toxin Type A free of complexing proteins in the treatment of blepharospasm. J Neural Transm (Vienna).; 113(3):303–312

[40] Comella CL, Jankovic J, Shannon KM, et al. Dystonia Study Group. Comparison of botulinum toxin serotypes A and B for the treatment of cervical dystonia. Neurology.; 65(9):1423–1429

[41] Pappert EJ, Germanson T, Myobloc/Neurobloc European Cervical Dystonia Study Group. Botulinum toxin type B vs. type A in toxin-naïve patients with cervical dystonia: Randomized, double-blind, noninferiority trial. Mov Disord.; 23(4):510–517

[42] Duarte GS, Castelão M, Rodrigues FB, et al. Botulinum toxin type A versus botulinum toxin type B for cervical dystonia. Cochrane Database Syst Rev.; 10:CD004314

[43] Brashear A, Bergan K, Wojcieszek J, Siemers ER, Ambrosius W. Patients' perception of stopping or continuing treatment of cervical dystonia with botulinum toxin type A. Mov Disord.; 15(1):150–153

[44] Jinnah HA, Comella CL, Perlmutter J, Lungu C, Hallett M, Dystonia Coalition Investigators. Longitudinal studies of botulinum toxin in cervical dystonia: Why do patients discontinue therapy? Toxicon.; 147:89–95

[45] Barnes MP, Best D, Kidd L, et al. The use of botulinum toxin type-B in the treatment of patients who have become unresponsive to botulinum toxin type-A – initial experiences. Eur J Neurol.; 12(12):947–955

[46] Jost WH, Benecke R, Hauschke D, et al. Clinical and pharmacological properties of incobotulinumtoxinA and its use in neurological disorders. Drug Des Devel Ther.; 9:1913–1926

[47] Tatu L, Jost WH. Anatomy and cervical dystonia: "Dysfunction follows form". J Neural Transm (Vienna).; 124(2):237–243

[48] Jost WH, Tatu L. Selection of muscles for botulinum toxin injections in cervical dystonia. Mov Disord Clin Pract (Hoboken).; 2(3):224–226

[49] Nijmeijer SW, Koelman JH, Kamphuis DJ, Tijssen MA. Muscle selection for treatment of cervical dystonia with botulinum toxin–a systematic review. Parkinsonism Relat Disord.; 18(6):731–736

[50] Comella CL, Buchman AS, Tanner CM, Brown-Toms NC, Goetz CG. Botulinum toxin injection for spasmodic torticollis: increased magnitude of benefit with electromyographic assistance. Neurology.; 42(4):878–882

[51] Schramm A, Bäumer T, Fietzek U, Heitmann S, Walter U, Jost WH. Relevance of sonography for botulinum toxin treatment of cervical dystonia: an expert statement. J Neural Transm (Vienna).; 122(10):1457–1463

[52] Anderson TJ, Rivest J, Stell R, et al. Botulinum toxin treatment of spasmodic torticollis. J R Soc Med.; 85(9):524–529

[53] Brashear A. Botulinum toxin type A in the treatment of patients with cervical dystonia. Biologics.; 3:1–7

[54] Benecke R, Dressler D. Botulinum toxin treatment of axial and cervical dystonia. Disabil Rehabil.; 29(23):1769–1777

8
Botulinum Neurotoxin for Hemifacial Spasm and Facial Synkinesis

Lesley French Childs, Daniel Novakovic, and Scott R. Gibbs

Summary

Hemifacial spasm is a disorder of recurrent, involuntary twitches of facial muscles that are peripherally induced. It typically begins in middle age and occurs more commonly in women. Most frequently, patients will experience involuntary eye closure and mouth retraction/elevation. The etiology is thought to be due to vascular compression of the facial nerve by an aberrant vascular loop, specifically the posterior inferior cerebellar artery. Botulinum neurotoxin is a safe, effective method to treat hemifacial spasm.

Keywords: hemifacial spasm, focal dystonia, botulinum neurotoxin

8.1 Introduction to Hemifacial Spasm

Hemifacial spasm is a disorder of recurrent, involuntary twitches of facial muscles that are peripherally induced. A disorder that typically begins in middle age and more commonly in women, hemifacial spasm often first involves the orbicularis oculi and spreads slowly to other facial muscles. There is a progression seen from increased blinking initially to forced closure of the eyelids. Later, twitching of the lower face can develop. The most common spasms include eye closure and mouth retraction/elevation. The likelihood of associated midfacial weakness increases with duration of the disorder. Although benign, this disorder affects patients both cosmetically and functionally. Unfortunately, the disorder is chronic, with only rare reports of spontaneous recovery. Defazio et al[1] described two patients in a series of 65 patients who experienced complete and long-lasting symptom relief during their second or third year of treatment with botulinum neurotoxin (BoNT). In a Cochrane review, only one randomized placebo-controlled trial involving 11 people was identified; this was performed by Yoshimura et al in 1992.[2] BoNT treatment was noted to be superior to treatment with a placebo. This, in combination with numerous other case series, suggests that BoNT is effective and safe for treating hemifacial spasm. The paucity of placebo-controlled trials comparing the efficacy of BoNT with placebo is likely due to the significant success of treatment with the toxin reported in open studies. Researchers would likely find it ethically difficult to randomize patients to simply examine efficacy. However, further trials to evaluate the technique of injection, dose, immunogenicity, and long-term efficacy would provide value.[3]

The etiology is thought to be due to vascular compression of the facial nerve by an aberrant vascular loop, specifically the posterior inferior cerebellar artery (PICA). Other causes of compression include tumors or vascular malformations. After vascular pressure has been exerted on the facial nerve, a secondary demyelination is thought to ensue. In contrast, a functional mechanical factor increasing nerve excitability is proposed by Lefaucheur,[4] stating this is due to compression or stretch resulting from the neurovascular conflict.

In an article investigating unusual causes of hemifacial spasm (other than vascular compression at the root exit zone of the facial nerve), Han et al[5] emphasized radiologic investigations for achieving accurate diagnoses. Specifically, cases of tumor compression, vascular malformation, and dolichoectatic vertebrobasilar arteries are discussed.

Treatment for hemifacial spasm includes oral doses of antiepileptic drugs (such as carbamazepine and baclofen as well as benzodiazepines), neurosurgical decompression of the seventh cranial nerve, or intramuscular BoNT injections. The BoNT injections obviate the need for oral medications, which have associated side effects and limited efficacy, as well as the risks associated with a major intracranial operation.[6] In the neurosurgical literature, a review on outcomes and complications in those undergoing microvascular decompression revealed a risk of permanent cranial nerve deficit of 1 to 2% for facial palsy, 2 to 3% for nonfunctional hearing loss, and 0.5 to 1% for lower cranial nerve dysfunction. Risk of stroke was at 0.1% and mortality at 0.1%. Cerebrospinal fluid leakage and related complications could be reduced by less than 2% in most series provided careful closing techniques are applied. Complications were at a higher rate in repeated microvascular decompression.[7] Because of the potential complications and the possibility of recurrence of spasms, most patients and physicians prefer using BoNT for long-term management of hemifacial spasm. Repeated treatments using Botox seem to maintain efficacy for treatment over a follow-up period of at least 10 years, based on level III evidence.[8] In fact, much evidence supports the use of BoNT as the first-line treatment for hemifacial spasm.[9]

Rudzińska et al[10] noted that the often-associated sensory and autonomic complaints of hemifacial spasm also responded to treatment with BoNT. Specifically, tearing, eye irritation, and a "clicking" sound (attributed to contractions of the stapedius muscle) were reduced after treatment with the toxin. This finding is likely due to the interference of transmission at the cholinergic synapses of the parasympathetic and postganglionic sympathetic nervous system.[10]

8.2 Introduction to Facial Synkinesis

One of the most troubling sequelae of facial nerve paralysis (most commonly resulting from tumor resection or from Bell's palsy) is synkinesis, which is the presence of unintentional motion in one area of the face produced during intentional movement in another area of the face. Of all the cranial nerves, the facial nerve is the most susceptible to traumatic injury due to its protracted course within the temporal bone. Synkinetic movements can be socially debilitating and can also be quite painful, with simultaneous spasm of multiple muscle groups. The most common form of synkinesis is oculo-oral, involving involuntary oral commissure movement with voluntary eye closure.

The etiology of synkinesis is thought to be multifactorial, with evidence supporting the role of aberrant axonal regeneration as well as central involvement in the form of facial nucleus hyperexcitability. Bajaj-Luthra et al[11] quantitatively analyzed the patterns of synkinetic facial movements on both the affected and unaffected sides. Patients with oculo-oral synkinesis were noted to have increased modiolar motion during eye closure relative to controls. (The modiolus is where several facial muscles converge toward a focus, just lateral to the buccal angle, to form a fibromuscular mass with three-dimensional mobility.) More specifically, in patients with synkinesis, the modiolar motion was noted to be asymmetric and increased in the horizontal and vertical planes. In consideration of both the affected and unaffected sides of the face, Neely et al[12] have described two types of synkinesis: synergistic synkinesis, in which movement on the affected side is similar to what might be seen on the unaffected side, but in excess thereof; and paradoxical synkinesis, in which the secondary facial movement is in a direction considered antagonistic to normal facial movement.

One of the earliest reported physiotherapy programs with consistent positive results for synkinesis rehabilitation is mime therapy, a technique developed in the Netherlands by collaboration between clinicians and mime actors.[13] Mirror technique whereby patients practice facial expressions in front of a mirror is a commonly employed biofeedback technique. Surgical treatment is also a possibility, and facial synkinesis manifests as zonal permutations of areas of "hyperkinesis and hypokinesis"; therefore, the surgical techniques that improve individ-

ual symptoms must aim to both restore and inhibit movement.[14]

The most common therapeutic modalities for the treatment of facial synkinesis include facial neuromuscular retraining and BoNT administration, which can augment the retraining and has a role as a salvage treatment for failed surgery.[15] In a study by Neville et al, the synkinesis assessment questionnaire (SAQ) scores were noted to decrease significantly for every question on the SAQ after treatment. The study also indicated that botulinum toxin type A (BTX-A) continues to be effective even after three rounds of treatment, with a significant decrease in overall scores after each treatment cycle.[16]

8.3 Workup

Hemifacial spasm needs to be distinguished from a focal dystonia (which is thought to be of central origin), as well as from blepharospasm (which is mostly bilateral), myokymia of the orbicularis oculi (which usually does not involve the lower face or cause complete eyelid closure), and synkinesis after Bell palsy. Thus, a thorough neurologic, ophthalmologic, and head and neck examination is crucial to accurately diagnose hemifacial spasm.

In patients with atypical features such as facial weakness, facial numbness, a decreased corneal reflex, or any other cranial nerve abnormalities, a space-occupying lesion should be excluded with magnetic resonance imaging/angiography. If such a lesion is identified, then neurosurgical consultation may provide benefit.

8.4 Anatomy

The patient sits comfortably upright or is placed in a reclining position. If lower facial injections are to be administered, electromyography (EMG) guidance is typically employed, and ground and reference electrodes are placed over the sternocleidomastoid muscle (SCM). The location of the desired injections should be marked on the skin, which is cleansed with an alcohol swab. Injections are administered using a 30- or 32-gauge needle or a hollow 27-gauge, Teflon-coated, monopolar EMG injection needle on a 1-mL tuberculin syringe. The orbicularis oculi injections are administered in the same manner as those for the treatment of blepharospasm (see Chapter 2). Treatment of the lower face is delayed until a response is achieved from the orbicularis oculi injections. In many cases, a periorbital injection to decrease the passive blink and the eye closure will also stop the mouth twitching and elevation. Usually, a reassessment at 2 weeks is needed before injecting the lower face.

The dose for the injections is typically 2.5 units (U)/0.1 mL of Botox (Botox, Allergan plc, Irvine, CA) in the pretarsal orbicularis oculi muscle (▶ Fig. 8.1) and also in the medial and lateral upper eyelid (▶ Fig. 8.2; ▶ Fig. 8.3), 2.5 U in the orbicularis oculi 1 cm from the lateral canthus (▶ Fig. 8.4), and 2.5 U in the lateral position of the inferior orbicularis oculi of the lower lid (▶ Fig. 8.5). The dose can be decreased for more mild symptoms. Patients with concurrent medial brow spasm may achieve further benefit from treatment of the procerus and corrugator supercilii muscles.

The procerus muscle is a pyramidal slip arising from the nasal bone and upper lateral cartilage that inserts into the skin between the eyebrows. Its purpose is to draw down the medial angle of the eyebrows, producing transverse rhytids over the bridge of the nose. The corrugator supercilii arises from the medial end of the superciliary arch. Its fibers pass

between the palpebral and orbital portions of the orbicularis oculi and insert into the deep surface of the skin, above the central orbital arch. The corrugator draws the eyebrow downward and medialward, producing vertical rhytids (▶ Fig. 8.5).[17]

For treatment of the lower face, 1.25 to 2.5 U can be injected under EMG control into the zygomaticus major, zygomaticus minor, levator anguli oris, depressor anguli oris, risorius, and platysma (▶ Fig. 8.5).

A brief review of these lower facial muscles is appropriate at this point, as a thorough understanding of facial anatomy is crucial for proper treatment technique. The zygomaticus major muscle arises from the zygomatic bone in front of the zygomaticotemporal suture. The muscle descends obliquely and inserts into the angle of the mouth. This muscle draws the angle of the mouth backward and upward, as in laughing. The zygomaticus minor originates from the malar bone and inserts into the outer portion of the upper lip. It draws the upper lip backward, upward, and outward.

The levator anguli oris arises from the canine fossa, just below the infraorbital foramen. These fibers insert into the angle of the mouth. The depressor anguli oris arises from the oblique line of the mandible and inserts into the angle of the mouth. The action of this muscle depresses the angle of the mouth, acting antagonistically to the action of the levator.

The risorius arises in the fascia over the masseter and passes horizontally forward, superficial to the platysma. It then inserts into the skin at the angle of the mouth. Its action retracts the angle of the mouth.

The platysma is a broad sheet arising from the fascia covering the upper parts of the pectoralis major and deltoid. The fibers cross the clavicle and proceed obliquely upward and medially along the

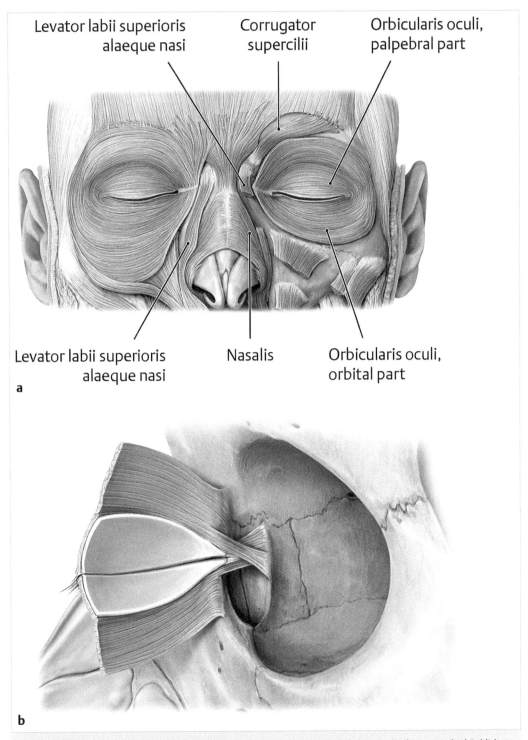

Levator labii superioris alaeque nasi

Corrugator supercilii

Orbicularis oculi, palpebral part

Levator labii superioris alaeque nasi

Nasalis

Orbicularis oculi, orbital part

a

b

Fig. 8.1 (a,b) Orbital anatomy. (From Gilroy AM et al. Atlas of Anatomy. 1st Ed. New York: Thieme Medical Publishers; 2008. Based on: Schuenke M, Schulte E, Schumacher U. THIEME Atlas of Anatomy: Head and Neuroanatomy. Illustrations by Voll M and Wesker K. 1st Ed. New York: Thieme Medical Publishers; 2008.)

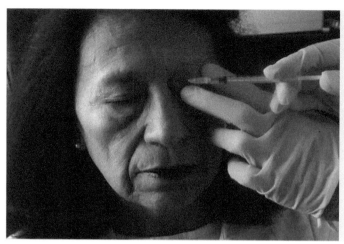

Fig. 8.2 Medial pretarsal orbicularis muscle injection.

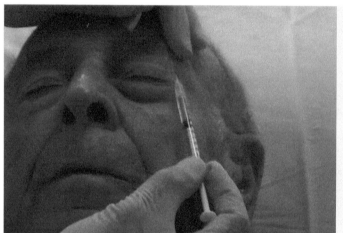

Fig. 8.3 Lateral pretarsal orbicularis muscle injection.

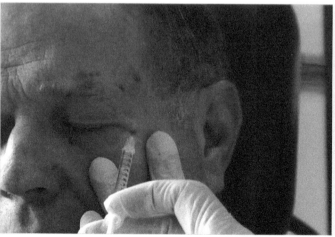

Fig. 8.4 Injection lateral to the lateral canthus.

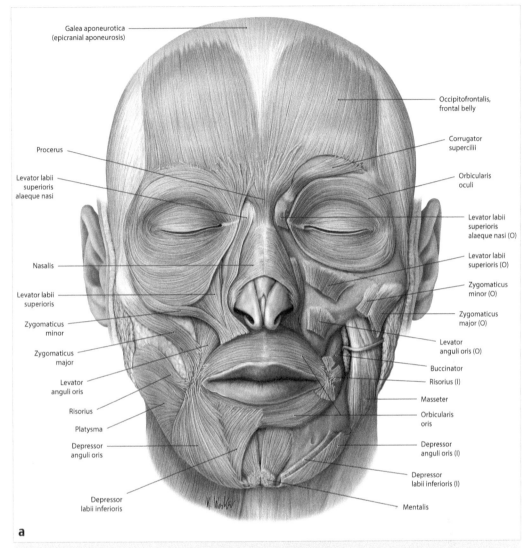

a

Fig. 8.5 **(a,b)** Muscles of facial expression. (From Gilroy AM et al. Atlas of Anatomy. 1st Ed. New York: Thieme Medical Publishers; 2008. Based on: Schuenke M, Schulte E, Schumacher U. THIEME Atlas of Anatomy: Head and Neuroanatomy. Illustrations by Voll M and Wesker K. 1st Ed. New York: Thieme Medical Publishers; 2008.) *(Continued)*

side of the neck. The anterior fibers interlace, below and behind the symphysis menti, with the fibers of the muscle of the opposite side; the posterior fibers cross the mandible, some being inserted into the bone below the oblique line, others into the skin and subcutaneous tissue of the lower part of the face, many of these fibers blending with the muscles

about the angle and lower part of the mouth. The platysma retracts and depresses the angle of the mouth.[17]

The doses used to treat synkinesis are typically lower than those used to treat hemifacial spasm, as the facial musculature is weaker at baseline. The goal is to weaken the abnormally stimulated muscles to allow for more symmetrical movement and

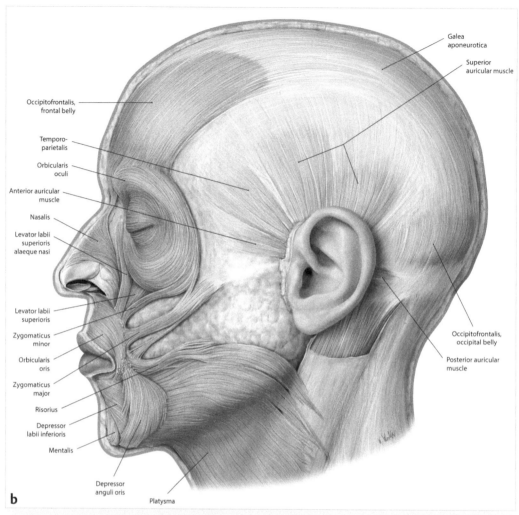

Galea
aponeurotica

Superior
auricular muscle

Occipitofrontalis,
frontal belly

Temporo-
parietalis

Orbicularis
oculi

Anterior auricular
muscle

Nasalis

Levator labii
superioris
alaeque nasi

Levator labii
superioris

Zygomaticus
minor

Orbicularis
oris

Zygomaticus
major

Risorius

Depressor
labii inferioris

Mentalis

Depressor
anguli oris

Platysma

Occipitofrontalis,
occipital belly

Posterior auricular
muscle

b

Fig. 8.5 (*Continued*) (**a,b**) Muscles of facial expression. (From Gilroy AM et al. Atlas of Anatomy. 1st Ed. New York: Thieme Medical Publishers; 2008. Based on: Schuenke M, Schulte E, Schumacher U. THIEME Atlas of Anatomy: Head and Neuroanatomy. Illustrations by Voll M and Wesker K. 1st Ed. New York: Thieme Medical Publishers; 2008.)

postures at rest. The upper and lower face is done at the same initial setting. Optimal dosing is decided on an individuated basis based on the patient's active and passive facial symmetry. The zygomaticus muscles, levator anguli oris, depressor anguli oris, risorius, and platysma are the most often injected muscles under EMG control.[6] Finally, contralateral facial musculature injections have value, as often the contralateral side of the face will compensate with hyperfunction resulting in eventual hypertrophy.[18]

8.5 Follow-up

Patients should return at 2 to 3 weeks for evaluation of the orbital effects and persistence of facial spasms. If additional injections of the orbicularis oculi are necessary, then further treatment can be administered at the follow-up visit. More commonly (to minimize side effects and adequately gauge response) additional treatment is deferred to the subsequent 3-month injection visit, when a higher total dose is utilized.[6]

8.6 Complications and Pitfalls

Complications include upper lid ptosis from diffusion of the toxin into the levator muscle. It is possible to help stimulate the muscle with a sympathomimetic eye drop such as apraclonidine 0.5 or 1.0% drops (1 drop t.i.d.). Exposure keratitis may result from a decreased blink, requiring artificial tear solution or a patch over the eye temporarily.

The nasolabial line may flatten from injections of the toxin, which may lead to an asymmetric smile, which may be corrected by smaller doses on future visits or injecting the normal side to lessen the disparity. Additionally, contour variations may be remedied by the injection of fillers.[6]

8.7 Conclusion

The successful treatment of hemifacial spasm and facial synkinesis affords an improved quality of life for patients, on both physical and emotional level. BoNT injections have proven to be a safe and effective treatment for these disorders and represent a preferable alternative to the other medical and surgical therapies currently available.

8.8 Key Points/Pearls

- Hemifacial spasm is a disorder of recurrent, involuntary twitches of facial muscles that are peripherally induced.
- The etiology of hemifacial spasm is most often due to vascular compression of the facial nerve by an aberrant vascular loop.
- Treatment options for hemifacial spasm include oral doses of antiepileptic drugs, neurosurgical decompression of the seventh cranial nerve, or intramuscular BoNT injections.
- BoNT injections for hemifacial spasm obviate the need for oral medications, with their associated side effects and limited efficacy, as well as the risks associated with a major intracranial operation.
- Facial synkinesis, a sequela of facial nerve paralysis, is the presence of unintentional motion in one area of the face produced during intentional movement in another area of the face.
- The etiology of synkinesis is thought to be multifactorial, with evidence supporting the role of aberrant axonal regeneration as well as central involvement in the form of facial nucleus hyperexcitability.
- The most common therapeutic modalities for the treatment of facial synkinesis include facial neuromuscular retraining and BoNT administration, which can augment the retraining.

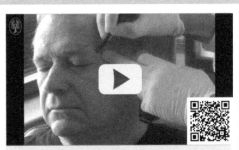

Video 8.1 Hemifacial spasm. Excessive function such as repetitive tight eye closure produces irritability and left hemifacial twitching. The most hyperfunctional areas of the patient's orbicularis oculi muscle are injected subcutaneously with 2.5 U/0.1 mL of Botox. For many patients, treating the eye and reducing spasms also quiets the midface. If not, the zygomaticus and levator labii superioris may also have to be treated. [1:25]

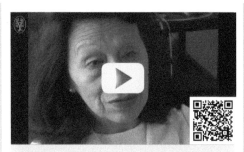

Video 8.2 Facial synkinesis. This patient has a post–Bell palsy left facial synkinesis. Notice her midface elevation on the left with eye closure. Her left orbicularis oculi muscle is injected in several places subcutaneously with 2.5 U/0.1 mL at each of the marked points. [3:02]

References

[1] Defazio G, Abbruzzese G, Girlanda P, et al. Botulinum toxin A treatment for primary hemifacial spasm: a 10-year multicenter study. Arch Neurol.; 59(3):418–420

[2] Yoshimura DM, Aminoff MJ, Tami TA, Scott AB. Treatment of hemifacial spasm with botulinum toxin. Muscle Nerve.; 15(9):1045–1049

[3] Costa J, Espírito-Santo C, Borges A, et al. Botulinum toxin type A therapy for hemifacial spasm. Cochrane Database Syst Rev. (1):CD004899

[4] Lefaucheur JP. New insights into the pathophysiology of primary hemifacial spasm. Neurochirurgie.; 64(2):87–93

[5] Han IB, Chang JH, Chang JW, Huh R, Chung SS. Unusual causes and presentations of hemifacial spasm. Neurosurgery.; 65(1):130–137, discussion 137

[6] Blitzer A, Brin MF. Management of hemifacial spasm and facial synkinesis with local injections of botulinum toxin. Otolaryngol Head Neck Surg.; 15:103–106

[7] Sindou M, Mercier P. Microvascular decompression for hemifacial spasm: Outcome on spasm and complications. A review. Neurochirurgie.; 64(2):106–116

[8] Bilyk JR, Yen MT, Bradley EA, Wladis EJ, Mawn LA. Chemodenervation for the Treatment of Facial Dystonia: A Report by the American Academy of Ophthalmology. Ophthalmology.; 125(9):1459–1467

[9] Kenney C, Jankovic J. Botulinum toxin in the treatment of blepharospasm and hemifacial spasm. J Neural Transm (Vienna).; 115(4):585–591

[10] Rudzińska M, Wójcik M, Szczudlik A. Hemifacial spasm non-motor and motor-related symptoms and their response to botulinum toxin therapy. J Neural Transm (Vienna).; 117(6):765–772

[11] Bajaj-Luthra A, VanSwearingen J, Thornton RH, Johnson PC. Quantitation of patterns of facial movement in patients with ocular to oral synkinesis. Plast Reconstr Surg.; 101(6):1473–1480

[12] Neely JG, Cheung JY, Wood M, Byers J, Rogerson A. Computerized quantitative dynamic analysis of facial motion in the paralyzed and synkinetic face. Am J Otol.; 13(2):97–107

[13] Beurskens CH, Heymans PG. Positive effects of mime therapy on sequelae of facial paralysis: stiffness, lip mobility, and social and physical aspects of facial disability. Otol Neurotol.; 24(4):677–681

[14] Markey JD, Loyo M. Latest advances in the management of facial synkinesis. Curr Opin Otolaryngol Head Neck Surg.; 25(4):265–272

[15] van Veen MM, Dusseldorp JR, Hadlock TA. Long-term outcome of selective neurectomy for refractory periocular synkinesis. Laryngoscope.; 128(10):2291–2295

[16] Neville C, Venables V, Aslet M, Nduka C, Kannan R. An objective assessment of botulinum toxin type A injection in the treatment of post-facial palsy synkinesis and hyperkinesis using the synkinesis assessment questionnaire. J Plast Reconstr Aesthet Surg.; 70(11):1624–1628

[17] Gray H. Anatomy of the Human Body, 20th ed. Philadelphia, PA: Lea & Febiger; 1918

[18] Markey JD, Loyo M. Latest advances in the management of facial synkinesis. Current Opinion in Otolaryngology & Head and Neck Surgery.; 25(4):265–272

9

Botulinum Neurotoxin for Hyperfunctional Facial Lines

Brian E. Benson, Diana N. Kirke, and Andrew Blitzer

Summary

There are many components to the ageing face; however, the most notable of these are hyperfunctional facial lines or rhytides. Botulinum neurotoxin (BoNT) has been shown to be a safe and effective temporary treatment of this condition in several prospective randomized controlled trials. As such, BoNT has been approved by the FDA as a temporary treatment for severe glabellar lines, moderate to severe lateral canthal lines/periocular lines, and for moderate to severe forehead lines and has thus become the most common nonsurgical aesthetic procedure. This chapter will discuss the workup of patients presenting for injection, the formulations of BoNT used, and the injection approach to each anatomic area of the face.

Keywords: botulinum toxin, hyperfunctional facial lines, rhytides

9.1 Introduction

Facial aging is a multifactorial process involving changes to skin, subcutaneous fat, muscle, and the underlying facial skeleton. Notable among these changes are hyperfunctional facial lines, rhytides, which develop with repetitive muscle activity. Over time, these lines deepen and remain apparent, even when the underlying musculature is relaxed. Both photodamage and smoking significantly accelerate these changes.

The ability of botulinum neurotoxin (BoNT) to reduce the appearance of facial lines was first noted in patients receiving treatment for hyperfunctional disorders such as hemifacial spasm and blepharospasm. Subsequent placebo-controlled studies confirmed the safety and efficacy of BoNT type A (BoNT-A) for the reduction of dynamic upper facial lines.[1,2] OnabotulinumtoxinA (Botox, Allergan plc, Irvine, CA) was approved by the United States Food and Drug Administration (FDA) in 2002 for the temporary treatment of moderate to severe glabellar lines, in 2013 for the temporary treatment of moderate to severe lateral canthal lines/periocular lines ("crow's feet"), and in 2017 for the temporary treatment of moderate to severe forehead lines associated with frontalis muscle activity. AbobotulinumtoxinA (Dysport; Ipsen Biopharmaceuticals Inc, Basking Ridge, NJ) and incobotulinumtoxinA (Xeomin; Merz Pharmaceuticals, Greensboro, NC) are currently approved only for the temporary treatment of moderate to severe glabellar lines. Data from the American Society for Aesthetic Plastic Surgery 2017 database indicate that treatment with BoNT-A for the reduction of facial lines is currently the most common nonsurgical aesthetic procedure in the United States, and its use has increased 30% during the 5-year survey period from 2012 to 2017. In 2017, a total of 1.55 million procedures were performed with BoNT-A and 722,394 procedures were performed with hyaluronic acid fillers, which together accounted for approximately 70% of all nonsurgical cosmetic procedures performed that year.[3]

There is now a substantial body of evidence supporting the safety and efficacy of BoNT-A for reduction of dynamic upper facial lines. However, extensive clinical experience has shown both BoNT-A and BoNT-B to be highly efficacious primary or adjunctive treatments of not just glabellar rhytides but also rhytides associated with hyperfunctional frontalis, orbicularis oculi, nasalis, orbicularis oris, depressor anguli oris, mentalis, and platysma muscles. It is also effective at reducing brow ptosis and the appearance of a hypertrophic pretarsal orbicularis oculi muscle.[4,5,6,7] In addition to the reduction of dynamic facial lines, recent research suggests that mild glabellar lines *in repose* are also reduced, although the mechanism of this "smoothing" phenomenon is not completely understood.[8] Paralysis of peri-incisional muscles with BoNT has also been shown to reduce facial scarring, especially in those lacerations perpendicular to relaxed skin tension lines.[9]

Reduction of dynamic facial lines may result in a more youthful appearance, as well as decreased inaccurate social interpretation of facial gestures suggesting anger or frustration. The goal of BoNT-A treatment is not only to reduce the appearance of rhytides but also to prevent the development of deep rhytides and thereby delay or avoid more invasive rejuvenation procedures. Based on an expanded facial rejuvenation paradigm incorporating three-dimensional volume restoration, BoNT-A is frequently used in conjunction with dermal fillers to meld facial movement control, recontouring, and volume enhancement to provide a more relaxed, youthful appearance.[4]

9.2 Workup

Patients should be interviewed regarding their medical history, medications, and prior cosmetic or reconstructive surgery. BoNT injection is contraindicated in patients with infection at the injection site, in patients with a known hypersensitivity to any ingredient in the formulation (including human albumin, saline, milk [abobotulinumtoxinA only]), in those receiving aminoglycosides, and in pregnant or lactating women. BoNT injection is relatively contraindicated in patients with disorders of the neuromuscular junction, myasthenia gravis, motor neuron disease, or Eaton-Lambert syndrome.[10] Furthermore, caution should be exercised in those patients with surgical alteration of facial anatomy, excessive dermatochalasis, and deep dermal scarring, as the effect of BoNT-A may be limited regarding the desired cosmetic outcome. Patients with active viral or bacterial illness have higher levels of circulating antibodies, which may decrease the efficacy of BoNT-A. Therefore, we recommend against BoNT-A injections in the setting of infection.

9.3 Botulinum Neurotoxin Formulations

Botulinum neurotoxin type A (Botox, Dysport, Xeomin) is approved for cosmetic use as discussed earlier. BoNT-B (Myobloc [rimabotulinumtoxinB]; Solstice Neurosciences, Inc., South San Francisco, CA) is not currently approved for cosmetic use. Although Botox/Dysport conversion ratios of 1:2.5, 1:3, and 1:4 have been reported in the literature, it is important to note that potency units for BoNT products are specific to each preparation, and are not interchangeable.[4] BoNT-B is generally considered less suitable for cosmetic use due to pain at the injection site due to low pH and shorter duration of effect.[4,11] Compared with Botox, Dysport may have a larger diffusion radius.[12]

9.3.1 General Considerations

Treatment planning and goals must be individualized according to specific anatomic variables including the location and depth of rhytids, size and position of facial musculature, brow position, eye shape, and skin type, as well as individual characteristic facial gestures and ethnic background. Examination during muscle activation as well as during repose is required to appreciate the contributions of the various muscles to facial rhytides. It should be noted that substantial differences exist between various ethnic aesthetic ideals. Therefore, additional treatment planning and customization may be required with different ethnic groups.

BoNT injections in patients older than 65 years frequently require additional modifications to accommodate thinner muscles and less robust fibroconnective tissue. Compared to younger patients, older patients are not likely to experience as significant of a reduction of rhytids with BoNT alone. Deeper facial lines resulting from soft-tissue changes and the long-term effects of gravity rather than hyperfunctional muscles frequently require additional volume enhancement and skin resurfacing interventions to achieve optimal results. Furthermore, older patients have a higher risk of bruising and migration of the toxin resulting in complications such as brow ptosis and blepharoptosis.[13] Clarifying goals, addressing anxieties, and dispelling misconceptions regarding the effects of BoNT-A are particularly important components of every consultation.

Most practitioners counsel the patient regarding the previously mentioned factors, as well as the role of dermal fillers in facial volume contouring, so that realistic goals and expectations may be established prior to initiating treatment with BoNT-A alone or in conjunction with other nonsurgical procedures. Although this chapter does not discuss volume contouring, the clinician is encouraged to become familiar with its use.

Doses are basic guidelines that should be modified based on individual anatomy, patient preference, and clinician judgment. For BoNT-A, the solution is reconstituted according to the standard formulation of 4 mL of saline per bottle, yielding 2.5 units (U) per 0.1 mL. These injections are typically performed using a 1.0-mL tuberculin syringe. An alternative reconstitution strategy is to use 1 mL of saline per 100-U bottle, yielding 1 U per 0.01 mL, injected with a 0.1-mL syringe. This technique creates smaller injection aliquots, which decreases the appearance of the bolus at the injection sites. The choice of the injection needle and syringe depends on the individual technique as well as on the specific application. Most practitioners use 29- to 32-gauge, ½- to 1¼-inch needles with 1-mL tuberculin syringes, 0.3-mL syringes, or 0.1-mL syringes (BD Medical, Franklin Lakes, NJ). The 0.1-mL syringes are particularly suited for use with the 1 U/0.01 mL dilution. Smaller gauge needles decrease injection pain, but become dull sooner, with subsequent loss of this advantage after multiple injections.

Although topical anesthesia is generally not required, some practitioners may use topical anesthetic such as lidocaine, ice, or massagers such as the Buzzy (MMJ Laboratories, Atlanta, GA) for vibration anesthesia in sensitive areas.[14] The depth of injection depends on the thickness of the skin, the amount of subcutaneous adipose tissue, and the size of the injected muscle. Most cosmetic injections do not require electromyographic (EMG) guidance, but it may be helpful in locating deeper or thinner muscles, such as the risorius or platysma.[10] Although there are no evidence-based guidelines, most practitioners massage the injection site after injection to produce hydrostatic pressure to facilitate some diffusion, but they instruct their patients to avoid manipulating these areas. Although contraction of the treated muscles has been shown to increase neurotoxin uptake, heavy physical exertion immediately after the injection is discouraged.

Complications of cosmetic BoNT-A injection can be grouped into three categories: local, locoregional, and systemic. Local complications include pain, erythema, ecchymosis, and hematoma formation. Locoregional complications are related to excessive weakening of facial and neck musculature or diffusion of the BoNT-A to adjacent muscles, resulting in brow ptosis, eyelid ptosis, facial asymmetry, oral incompetence, dysarthria, and dysphagia. These complications are dose and technique related, and may be avoided by injection of small volumes and using EMG guidance, when necessary. Systemic complications, including fatigue, generalized weakness, and nausea, are extremely rare, even when larger doses are used.[4] However, patients who receive large and frequent doses are at risk for developing neutralizing antibodies to the toxin, which will render the patient resistant to future BoNT-A therapy.[15]

9.3.2 Horizontal Forehead Lines

Anatomy

The frontalis muscle elevates the brows and the skin of the forehead, resulting in horizontal lines often associated with aging (▶ Fig. 9.1, ▶ Fig. 9.2, ▶ Table 9.1).

Although BoNT-A injection of the frontalis muscle reduces the appearance of horizontal facial lines, if used without concurrent injection of the brow depressors (see section "Glabellar Lines"), it may have the undesirable effect of lowering the brows.

Technique

Four to eight points (1.5–2.5 U BoNT-A per point) are injected in a curved horizontal line or two rows for a large forehead, crossing both the medial and lateral fibers at least 1.5 cm above the brow (▶ Fig. 9.3). Most practitioners now inject less BoNT-A in the frontalis muscle than they did in the past, thereby avoiding the "frozen face" look associated with paralysis of the frontalis muscle. Rather than immobilization, the goal of treatment should be a more relaxed, natural appearance. Typical starting doses for women range between 6 and 15 U, with men usually requiring higher doses of 6 to greater than 15 U.

Follow-up

If inadequate correction of horizontal forehead rhytids or overarching of the brows is noted, then additional BoNT-A may be injected a minimum of 7 days after the initial injections, at which time the expected effect of the initial BoNT-A should be achieved.

Complications

Keep in mind that the frontalis muscle is a brow elevator; so, keep the injection sites well above the brow and keep doses low to decrease the risk of brow ptosis. Doses greater than 20 U are more likely to result in complications. Brow ptosis may be managed with an additional corrugator injection or injection of the depressor supercilii directly below the brow.

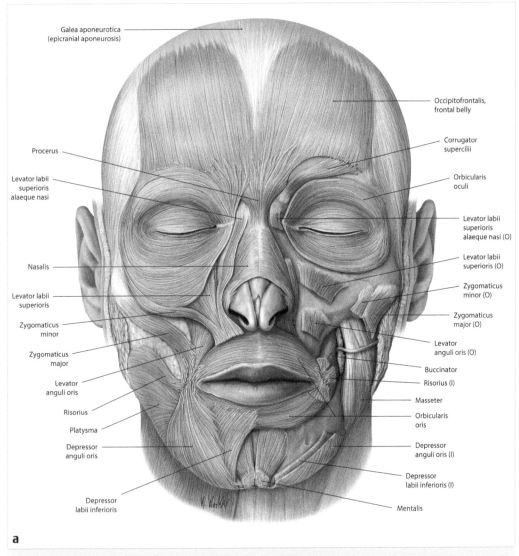

Fig. 9.1 (a,b) Muscles of facial expression. (From Gilroy AM et al. Atlas of Anatomy. 1st Ed. New York: Thieme Medical Publishers; 2008. Based on: Schuenke M, Schulte E, Schumacher U. THIEME Atlas of Anatomy: Head and Neuroanatomy. Illustrations by Voll M and Wesker K. 1st Ed. New York: Thieme Medical Publishers; 2008.) (*Continued*)

The medial fibers of the frontalis are usually stronger than the lateral fibers. Isolated injection of the medial fibers can result in the overarched "Spock eyebrow" caused by unopposed lateral fiber compensation to medial fiber injection. This phenomenon may also be seen following glabellar injections, whereby the weakened brow depressors, the corrugator and procerus, are unable to counteract the unopposed lateral frontal fibers. Low-dose injections to the upper lateral frontalis muscle will correct this undesirable effect.

Upper eyelid ptosis (blepharoptosis) may occur if the lateral injection is performed too close to the eyebrow, and diffusion occurs into the levator palpebral superioris. This phenomenon may be avoided by applying digital pressure below the injection site

93

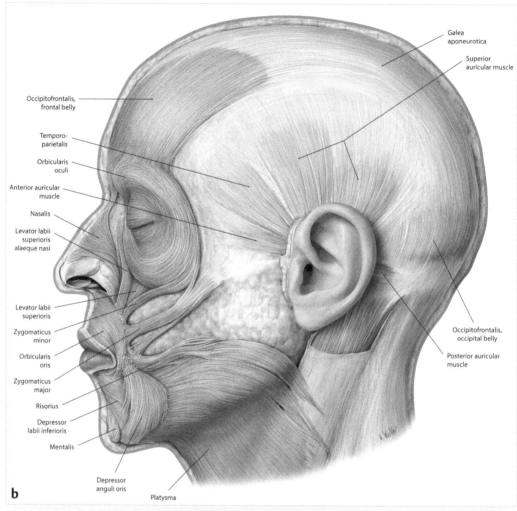

Galea
aponeurotica

Superior
auricular muscle

Occipitofrontalis,
frontal belly

Temporo-
parietalis

Orbicularis
oculi

Anterior auricular
muscle

Nasalis

Levator labii
superioris
alaeque nasi

Levator labii
superioris

Zygomaticus
minor

Orbicularis
oris

Zygomaticus
major

Risorius

Depressor
labii inferioris

Mentalis

Occipitofrontalis,
occipital belly

Posterior auricular
muscle

b

Depressor
anguli oris

Platysma

Fig. 9.1 (*Continued*) (**a,b**) Muscles of facial expression. (From Gilroy AM et al. Atlas of Anatomy. 1st Ed. New York: Thieme Medical Publishers; 2008. Based on: Schuenke M, Schulte E, Schumacher U. THIEME Atlas of Anatomy: Head and Neuroanatomy. Illustrations by Voll M and Wesker K. 1st Ed. New York: Thieme Medical Publishers; 2008.)

to prevent migration of the bolus. Should blepharoptosis occur, it may be partially ameliorated with apraclonidine or phenylephrine ophthalmic drops, which stimulate Mueller muscle to elevate the upper eyelid. Most cases of blepharoptosis are mild to moderate and resolve within 2 to 3 weeks.[16]

9.3.3 Glabellar Lines

Anatomy

The glabellar complex is composed of the procerus, corrugator supercilii, depressor

supercilii, and orbicularis oculi, all of which are brow depressors (▶ Fig. 9.1, ▶ Fig. 9.4). The corrugator supercilii also draws the brows medially, resulting in vertical glabellar lines. Different glabellar "frown patterns" may occur, depending on the relative contribution of the vertical and horizontal vectors.

Technique

Five to seven injection points are identified in a **V**-shaped pattern, with the narrow

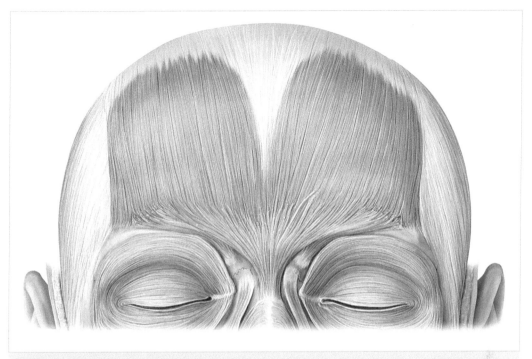

Fig. 9.2 Occipitofrontalis muscle. (From Gilroy AM et al. Atlas of Anatomy. 1st Ed. New York: Thieme Medical Publishers; 2008. Based on: Schuenke M, Schulte E, Schumacher U. THIEME Atlas of Anatomy: Head and Neuroanatomy. Illustrations by Voll M and Wesker K. 1st Ed. New York: Thieme Medical Publishers; 2008.)

point immediately cranial to the insertion of the procerus muscle at the nasion. A total of 10 to 30 U is commonly used in women and 20 to 40 U in men. As with frontalis injections, most clinicians now inject less than they did in the past. To avoid inadvertent injection into the frontalis, the upper injections should be placed no more than 1 cm superior to the orbital rim. To avoid brow ptosis, injection lateral to the midpupillary line should be avoided (▶ Fig. 9.5).

Follow-up

If inadequate correction of glabellar rhytids or overarching of the brows is noted, additional BoNT-A may be injected a minimum of 7 days after the initial injections, at which time the expected effect of the initial BoNT-A should be achieved.

Complications

Excessive or asymmetric elevation of the lateral brow, or "Spock eyebrow," can occur, whereby the weakened brow depressors, the corrugator and procerus, are unable to counteract the unopposed lateral frontal fibers. The management of this problem is low-dose injections (1–2.5 U) to the middle or lower lateral frontalis muscle. Patients with narrow brows should receive fewer injections and lower doses than patients with broad brows.

Upper eyelid ptosis (blepharoptosis) may occur if the injections are performed too close to the eyebrow, and diffusion occurs into the levator palpebral superioris. This phenomenon may be avoided by grasping the corrugator muscle during injection or by applying digital pressure below the injection site to prevent migration of the bolus. Blepharoptosis may be partially ameliorated with apraclonidine

Table 9.1 Muscles of facial expression: forehead, nose, and ear

Muscle	Origin	Insertion[a]	Main action(s)[b]
Calvaria			
1. Occipitofrontalis (frontal belly)	Epicranial aponeurosis	Skin and subcutaneous tissue of eyebrows and forehead	Elevates eyebrows, wrinkles skin of forehead
Palpebral fissure and nose			
2. Procerus	Nasal bone, lateral nasal cartilage (upper part)	Skin of lower forehead between eyebrows	Pulls medial angle of eyebrows inferiorly, producing transverse wrinkles over bridge of nose
3. Orbicularis oculi	Medial orbital margin, medial palpebral ligament, lacrimal bone	Skin around margin of orbit, superior and inferior tarsal plates	Acts as orbital sphincter (closes eyelids) • Palpebral portion gently closes • Orbital portion tightly closes (as in winking)
4. Nasalis	Maxilla (superior region of canine ridge)	Nasal cartilages	Flares nostrils by drawing ala (side) of nose toward nasal septum
5. Levator labii superioris alaeque nasi	Maxilla (frontal process)	Alar cartilage of nose and upper lip	Elevates upper lip, opens nostril
Ear			
6. Anterior auricular muscles	Temporal fascia (anterior portion)	Helix of the ear	Pull ear superiorly and anteriorly
7. Superior auricular muscles	Epicranial aponeurosis on side of head	Upper portion of auricle	Elevate ear
8. Posterior auricular muscles	Mastoid process	Convexity of concha of ear	Pull ear superiorly and posteriorly

Source: Adapted with permission from Schuenke M, Schulte E, Schumacher U. THIEME Atlas of Anatomy: Head and Neuroanatomy. New York, NY: Thieme; 2008:47.
[a]There are no bony insertions for the muscles of facial expression.
[b]All muscles of facial expression are innervated by the facial nerve (cranial nerve VII) via temporal, zygomatic, buccal, mandibular, or cervical branches arising from the parotid plexus.

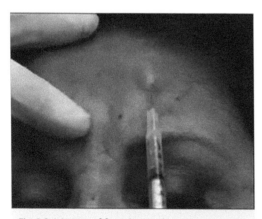

Fig. 9.3 Injection of frontalis muscle.

or phenylephrine ophthalmic drops, which stimulate Mueller muscle to elevate the upper eyelid. Most cases of blepharoptosis are mild to moderate and resolve within 2 to 3 weeks.[6,16]

9.3.4 Brow Lift

Hyperfunction of the brow depressors results in a lowered brow, a facial gesture that may be associated with emotional states such as anger, fatigue, frustration, and anxiety. The concept of the "Botox brow lift" is based on selective weakening

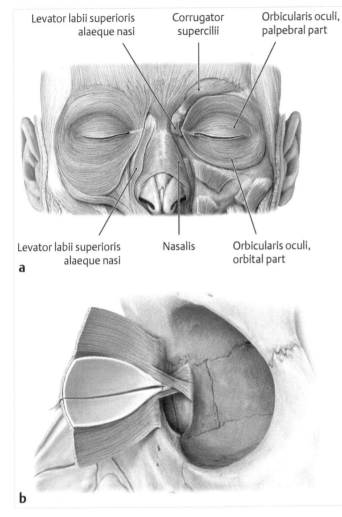

Levator labii superioris alaeque nasi

Corrugator supercilii

Orbicularis oculi, palpebral part

Levator labii superioris alaeque nasi

Nasalis

Orbicularis oculi, orbital part

a

Fig. 9.4 (a,b) Muscles of facial expression in the periorbital anatomy. (From Gilroy AM et al. Atlas of Anatomy. 1st Ed. New York: Thieme Medical Publishers; 2008. Based on: Schuenke M, Schulte E, Schumacher U. THIEME Atlas of Anatomy: Head and Neuroanatomy. Illustrations by Voll M and Wesker K. 1st Ed. New York: Thieme Medical Publishers; 2008.)

b

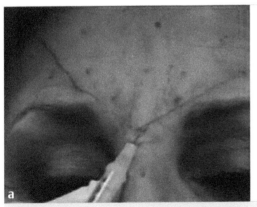
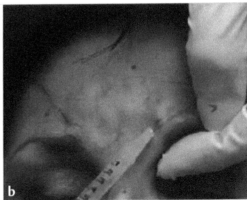

a

b

Fig. 9.5 (a,b) Injection of the glabellar complex.

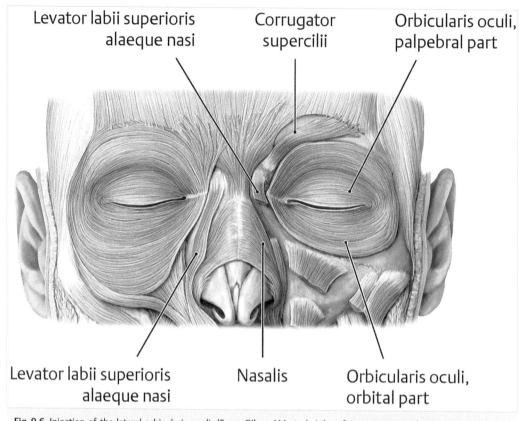

Levator labii superioris alaeque nasi

Corrugator supercilii

Orbicularis oculi, palpebral part

Levator labii superioris alaeque nasi

Nasalis

Orbicularis oculi, orbital part

Fig. 9.6 Injection of the lateral orbicularis oculi. (From Gilroy AM et al. Atlas of Anatomy. 1st Ed. New York: Thieme Medical Publishers; 2008. Based on: Schuenke M, Schulte E, Schumacher U. THIEME Atlas of Anatomy: Head and Neuroanatomy. Illustrations by Voll M and Wesker K. 1st Ed. New York: Thieme Medical Publishers; 2008.)

of the brow depressors, resulting in unopposed brow elevation by the frontalis-muscle. Several investigators have documented 1- to 4.8-mm elevation of the brow following injection of the brow depressors or medial frontalis fibers. This effect may be achieved with the traditional glabellar injection pattern (▶ Fig. 9.5), but may also be augmented by lateral orbicularis oculi injections performed below the brow, but superior and lateral to the orbital rim (▶ Fig. 9.6). As mentioned earlier, selective weakening of the medial frontalis fibers may also result in increased resting tone of the lateral fibers, thereby resulting in elevation of the middle and lateral brow. These techniques are also useful for those patients with eyebrow asymmetry as a result of trauma, surgery, and facial nerve paralysis.

9.3.5 Periocular Lines ("Crow's Feet")

Anatomy

The orbicularis oculi muscle originates from the nasal process of the frontal bone, the lacrimal bone, and the medial palpebral ligament. It is divided into three concentric portions: lacrimal (innermost), palpebral, and orbital (outermost) (▶ Fig. 9.4). The fibers of the orbital portion form a complete ellipse around the eye, with the outermost fibers blending with the frontalis, corrugator, and masseter. Contraction of the lateral orbital fibers of the orbicularis oculi results in the characteristic radial periocular lines known as "crow's feet." These rhytides frequently develop earlier in fair-skinned individuals, smokers, and those with photodamage.

Technique

Two to five injection sites no closer than 1 cm lateral to the lateral orbital rim are used to inject a total of 10 to 30 U in women and 20 to 30 U in men (▶ Fig. 9.7). Many experienced clinicians are now injecting increased amounts of BoNT-A in men. These injections are frequently used in combination with malar volume augmentation.

Follow-up

If inadequate correction of periocular lines is noted, additional BoNT-A may be injected a minimum of 7 days after the initial injections, at which time the expected effect of the initial BoNT-A should be achieved.

Complications

Special care must be paid to avoid disrupting the small superficial blood vessels in the periorbital region. Placing the patient in a prone position and using proper lighting will help the injector to avoid bruising. Superficial deep dermal injections rather than intramuscular injection may also reduce the risk of bruising.

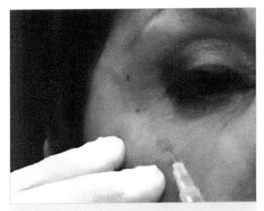

Fig. 9.7 Injection of the orbicularis oculi muscle.

Extensive preinjection counseling regarding the minimal effect on deep lines, upper eyelid hooding, and lower lid changes best treated with fillers, skin resurfacing techniques, or surgery is critically important to avoid unrealistic patient expectations regarding BoNT-A treatment in this dynamic, complex anatomic region.[17]

9.3.6 Hypertrophic Pretarsal Orbicularis

Anatomy

Smiling decreases the perceived size of the palpebral aperture. Some patients seek a more rounded-appearing eye, both at rest and during smiling. The practitioner can achieve this appearance by injecting the inferior pretarsal orbicularis oculi muscle (▶ Fig. 9.8). These injections also decrease lower eyelid fine lines, but not deep lines or dermatochalasis.

Technique

These injections are administered subcutaneously along the tarsal plate. The patient is asked to look up, and the needle is placed several millimeters below the lash line (▶ Fig. 9.9). The injections should not be given any more medial than the midpapillary line to prevent epiphora from too much orbicularis weakening. No more than 2 U of BoNT-A should be injected per eyelid.

Follow-up

If inadequate correction of the hypertrophic pretarsal orbicularis is noted, additional BoNT-A may be injected a minimum of 7 days after the initial injections, at which time the expected effect of the initial BoNT-A should be achieved.

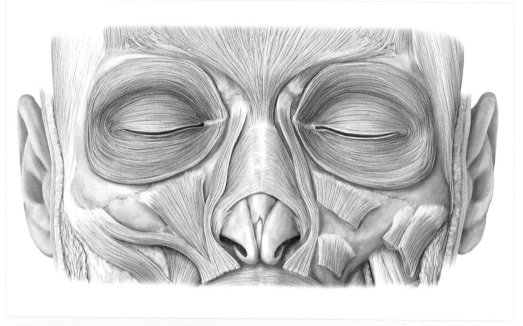

Fig. 9.8 Orbicularis oculi muscle. (From Gilroy AM et al. Atlas of Anatomy. 1st Ed. New York: Thieme Medical Publishers; 2008. Based on: Schuenke M, Schulte E, Schumacher U. THIEME Atlas of Anatomy: Head and Neuroanatomy. Illustrations by Voll M and Wesker K. 1st Ed. New York: Thieme Medical Publishers; 2008.)

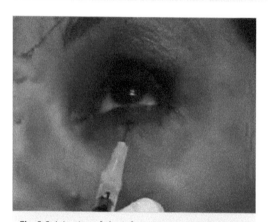

Fig. 9.9 Injection of the inferior pretarsal orbicularis oculi muscle.

Complications

Care must be taken to avoid small vessels to prevent bruising. These injections should not be given to patients who fail the "snap test" to evaluate laxity of the tarsal plate, patients who have had lower eyelid ablative resurfacing, or patients with dry eyes or scleral show.[7]

9.3.7 Nasalis ("Bunny Lines")

Anatomy

"Bunny lines" are dynamic vertically oriented rhytids on the lateral aspect of the nasal dorsum that may extend to the lower eyelids and cheeks when the patient smiles or laughs. These lines result from the contraction of the nasalis muscle, which is a U-shaped muscle with transverse fibers extending across the nasal dorsum, and vertical fibers running down the lateral dorsum (▶ Fig. 9.4). These fibers move the nose and control the size of the nostrils.

Technique

A dose of 2.5 to 5 U is injected into the midportion of the nasalis muscle, which is located halfway between the dorsum of the nose and the face of the maxilla over the nasal bone (▶ Fig. 9.10).

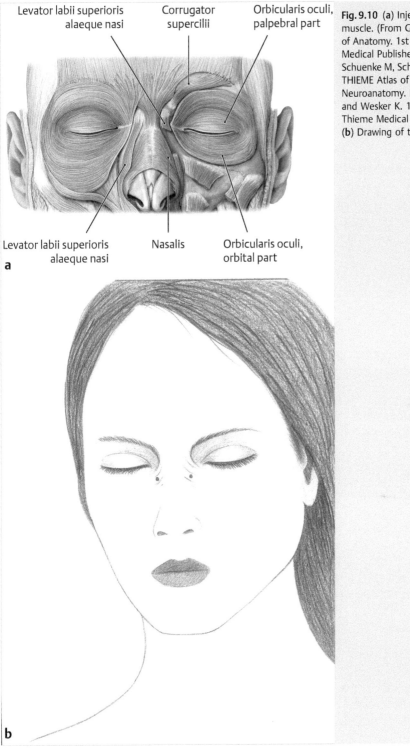

Levator labii superioris alaeque nasi

Corrugator supercilii

Orbicularis oculi, palpebral part

Levator labii superioris alaeque nasi

Nasalis

Orbicularis oculi, orbital part

a

b

Fig. 9.10 (a) Injection of the nasalis muscle. (From Gilroy AM et al. Atlas of Anatomy. 1st Ed. New York: Thieme Medical Publishers; 2008. Based on: Schuenke M, Schulte E, Schumacher U. THIEME Atlas of Anatomy: Head and Neuroanatomy. Illustrations by Voll M and Wesker K. 1st Ed. New York: Thieme Medical Publishers; 2008.) (b) Drawing of the injection sites.

Follow-up

If inadequate correction of nasalis lines is noted, then additional BoNT-A may be injected a minimum of 7 days after the initial injections, at which time the expected effect of the initial BoNT-A should be achieved.

Complications

Pain at the injection sites and bruising may occur. The clinician must keep volumes small to prevent diffusion to the medial rectus muscle, levator labii superioris, or the levator labii alaeque nasi.[7,17]

9.3.8 Perioral Lines

Anatomy

The orbicularis oris is a sphincter muscle whose fibers mediate the closure and protrusion of the lips (▶ Fig. 9.11; ▶ Table 9.2). Perioral lines, also called "smoker's lines" or "lipstick lines," result from pleating of the skin during contraction of the orbicularis oris muscle.

Technique

Low-dose injections are given on each side of the upper lip, 5 to 8 mm above the mucocutaneous junction (▶ Fig. 9.12). A total of two or four injections may be administered, with a total of 2 to 5 U, depending on the horizontal length of the lip and the severity of the lines. These lines can also be treated with small amounts of filler agents, or laser or chemical peels in the areas of the deepest lines.

Follow-up

If inadequate correction of perioral lines is noted, additional BoNT-A may be injected a minimum of 7 days after the initial injections, at which time the expected effect of the initial BoNT-A should be achieved.

Complications

Only small amounts of toxin should be given or else patients will develop lip incompetence, drooling, or dysarthria. The lateral injection points should be at least 1.5 cm away from the oral commissure. These injections are relatively contraindicated in professional singers, actors, and wind instrumentalists.[17]

9.3.9 Excessive Gingival Display ("Gummy Smile")

Anatomy

Excessive gingival display is related to hyperfunction of the levator labii superioris alaeque nasalis, levator labii superioris, levator anguli oris, zygomaticus major and minor, and the depressor septi nasi muscles in conjunction with individual anatomic characteristics such as size and configuration of the upper lip and maxilla.

Technique

Due to the complex interplay of these muscles, conservative treatment is aimed at weakening the levator labii superioris alaeque nasalis muscle, by injecting 1 to 2.5 U at the inferior edge of the nasal bone at the junction of the maxilla. An alternative treatment target is the depressor septi nasi, which is injected with 2 to 3 U at the base of the columella (▶ Fig. 9.13).

Follow-up

If inadequate correction of excessive gingival display is noted, then additional BoNT-A may be injected a minimum of 7 days after the initial injections, at which time the expected effect of the initial BoNT-A should be achieved.

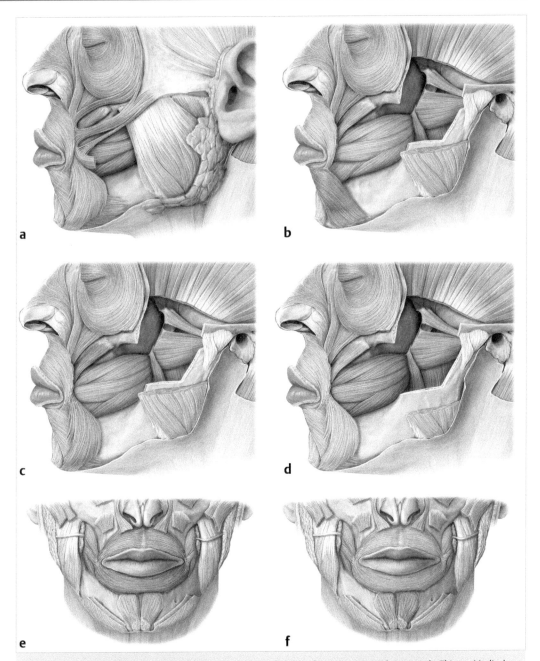

Fig. 9.11 (a–f) Muscles of the mouth. (From Gilroy AM et al. Atlas of Anatomy. 1st Ed. New York: Thieme Medical Publishers; 2008. Based on: Schuenke M, Schulte E, Schumacher U. THIEME Atlas of Anatomy: Head and Neuroanatomy. Illustrations by Voll M and Wesker K. 1st Ed. New York: Thieme Medical Publishers; 2008.)

Table 9.2 Muscles of facial expression: mouth and neck

Muscle	Origin	Insertion[a]	Main action(s)[b]
Mouth			
1. Zygomaticus major	Zygomatic bone (lateral surface)	Skin at corner of the mouth	Pulls corner of mouth superiorly and laterally
2. Zygomaticus minor	Zygomatic bone (posterior part)	Upper lip just medial to corner of the mouth	Pulls upper lip superiorly
3. Levator labii superioris alaeque nasi	Maxilla (frontal process)	Alar cartilage of nose and upper lip	Elevates upper lip, opens nostril
4. Levator labii superioris	Maxilla (frontal process) and infraorbital region	Skin of upper lip, alar cartilages of nose	Elevates upper lip, dilates nostril, raises angle of the mouth
5. Depressor labii inferioris	Mandible (anterior portion of oblique line)	Lower lip at midline; blends with muscle from opposite side	Pulls lower lip inferiorly and laterally
6. Levator anguli oris	Maxilla (below infraorbital foramen)	Skin at corner of the mouth	Raises angle of the mouth, helps form nasolabial furrow
7. Depressor anguli oris	Mandible (oblique line below canine, premolar, and first molar teeth)	Skin at corner of the mouth; blends with orbicularis oris	Pulls angle of the mouth inferiorly and laterally
8. Buccinator	Mandible, alveolar processes of maxilla and mandible, pterygomandibular raphe	Angle of mouth, orbicularis oris	Presses cheek against molar teeth, working with tongue to keep food between occlusal surfaces and out of oral vestibule; expels air from oral cavity/resists distension when blowing *Unilateral:* draws mouth to one side
9. Orbicularis oris	Deep surface of skin Superiorly: maxilla (median plane) Inferiorly: mandible	Mucous membrane of lips	Acts as oral sphincter • Compresses and protrudes lips (e.g., when whistling, sucking, and kissing) • Resists distension (when blowing)
Risorius	Fascia over masseter	Skin of corner of the mouth	Retracts corner of mouth as in grimacing
10. Mentalis	Mandible (incisive fossa)	Skin of chin	Elevates and protrudes lower lip
Neck			
11. Platysma	Skin over lower neck and upper lateral thorax	Mandible (inferior border), skin over lower face, angle of the mouth	Depresses and wrinkles skin of lower face; tenses skin of neck; aids in forced depression of the mandible

Source: Adapted with permission from Schuenke M, Schulte E, Schumacher U. THIEME Atlas of Anatomy: Head and Neuroanatomy. New York, NY: Thieme; 2008:47.
[a]There are no bony insertions for the muscles of facial expression.
[b]All muscles of facial expression are innervated by the facial nerve (cranial nerve VII) via temporal, zygomatic, buccal, mandibular, or cervical branches arising from the parotid plexus.

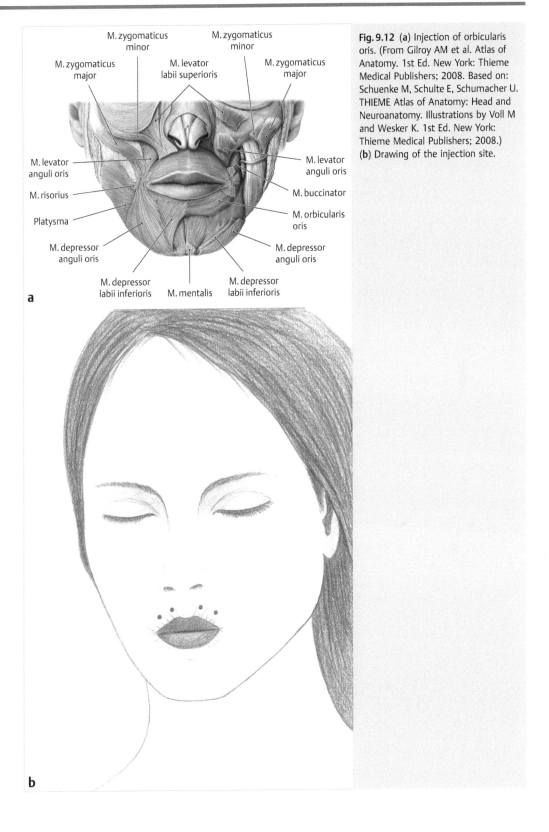

M. zygomaticus minor

M. zygomaticus minor

M. zygomaticus major

M. levator labii superioris

M. zygomaticus major

M. levator anguli oris

M. levator anguli oris

M. risorius

M. buccinator

Platysma

M. orbicularis oris

M. depressor anguli oris

M. depressor anguli oris

M. depressor labii inferioris

M. mentalis

M. depressor labii inferioris

a

b

Fig. 9.12 (a) Injection of orbicularis oris. (From Gilroy AM et al. Atlas of Anatomy. 1st Ed. New York: Thieme Medical Publishers; 2008. Based on: Schuenke M, Schulte E, Schumacher U. THIEME Atlas of Anatomy: Head and Neuroanatomy. Illustrations by Voll M and Wesker K. 1st Ed. New York: Thieme Medical Publishers; 2008.) (b) Drawing of the injection site.

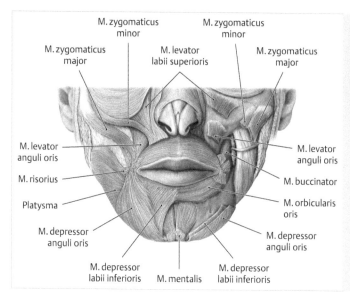

Fig. 9.13 Muscles of the lower face. (From Gilroy AM et al. Atlas of Anatomy. 1st Ed. New York: Thieme Medical Publishers; 2008. Based on: Schuenke M, Schulte E, Schumacher U. THIEME Atlas of Anatomy: Head and Neuroanatomy. Illustrations by Voll M and Wesker K. 1st Ed. New York: Thieme Medical Publishers; 2008.)

Complications

Too much toxin will cause too much weakness of the levator system and can result in upper lip ptosis, smile asymmetry, and excessive lengthening of the upper lip. These injections are relatively contraindicated in professional singers, actors, and wind instrumentalists as well.[17,18]

9.3.10 Melomental Folds ("Marionette Lines")

Anatomy

Melomental folds are vertical lines that extend from the modiolus to the lateral mentum due to the downward pull of the triangular-shaped depressor anguli oris (DAO) muscles (▶ Fig. 9.11c, ▶ Table 9.2). Although they may be treated with soft-tissue augmentation alone, the addition of BoNT-A will extend the life of the augmentation and decrease the unhappy appearance of the downward turned lip.

Technique

The patient is asked to pull the lower lip in a downward direction so that the DAO

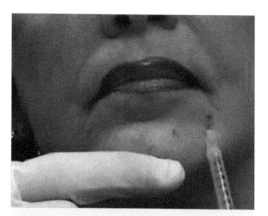

Fig. 9.14 Injection of the depressor anguli oris.

can be palpated. It should be injected with 5 U of BoNT-A at the midpoint between the lip edge and the lower border of the mandible (▶ Fig. 9.14). If the injection is placed too high, then there may be significant weakening of the orbicularis oris.

Follow-up

If inadequate correction of melomental folds is noted, additional BoNT-A may be injected a minimum of 7 days after the initial injections, at which time the expected effect of the initial BoNT-A should be achieved.

Complications

If the injection is placed too high, drooling and dysarthria can result from weakening of the orbicularis oris. These injections are relatively contraindicated in professional singers, actors, and wind instrumentalists.[17]

9.3.11 Mental Crease and "Peau d'orange"

Anatomy

The mentalis is a perpendicular muscle that covers the chin and inserts transversely in the dermis of the lower lip (▶ Fig. 9.11f, ▶ Table 9.2). Contraction of the mentalis can produce a prominent mental crease or the dimpled appearance termed "*peau d'orange.*" These findings may be increasingly noticeable as the subcutaneous fat and dermal collagen is lost over time.

Technique

A total of 4 to 5 U in women and 6 to 10 U in men are injected either with one midline injection or bilaterally in the lower third of the mentalis muscles (▶ Fig. 9.15). BoNT-A treatment may be combined with fillers with good effect.

Follow-up

If inadequate correction of the mental crease or *peau d'orange* is noted, then additional BoNT-A may be injected a minimum of 7 days after the initial injections, at which time the expected effect of the initial BoNT-A should be achieved.

Complications

If the injection is placed above the mental crease, then there may be weakening of the orbicularis oris producing drooling or dysarthria.[10,17]

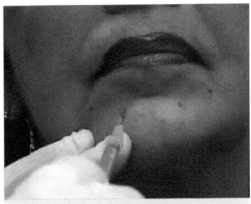

Fig. 9.15 Injection of the mentalis muscle.

9.3.12 Vertical Platysmal Bands

Anatomy

These vertical neck bands are caused by the edge of a hyperactive platysma muscle. The platysma is a thin, broad muscle that originates from the border of the mandible/ SMAS (superficial musculo-aponeurotic system) and inserts in the clavicular region (▶ Fig. 9.1). These bands are most prominent during smiling, speaking, or other social gestures. Their appearance may be exaggerated after a face-lift, especially if platysmal plication is not performed.

Technique

The anterior border and posterior borders of the muscles are outlined on the skin. Sequential horizontal lines are drawn starting approximately 1 cm below the mandible, and repeated every 1.5 cm. Either small amounts (2.5 U per 0.1 mL) are given directly into the edge of the platysma every 1 to 2 cm, or, using EMG guidance, the muscle can be entered along the long axis, and then injected as the needle is withdrawn (▶ Fig. 9.16). Usually, a total of 10 to 15 U per muscle is administered.

Follow-up

If inadequate correction of vertical platysmal bands is noted, then additional

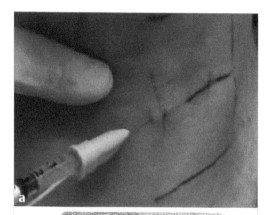

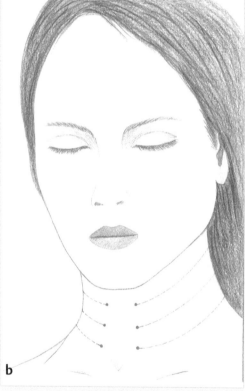

Fig. 9.16 (a) Injection of the platysma muscle; (b) drawing of the injection site.

BoNT-A may be injected a minimum of 7 days after the initial injections, at which time the expected effect of the initial BoNT-A should be achieved.

Complications

If too much toxin is given, or if the BoNT-A is injected too deeply, the strap muscles may be weakened. This may result in poor elevation of the larynx with swallowing, thereby producing dysphagia. The most important area to avoid is the cervicomental junction, due to the close proximity of the swallowing musculature. The toxin may also migrate medially to the cricothyroid muscle, causing pitch changes during voicing.[10]

9.3.13 Horizontal Platysmal Bands ("Necklace Bands")

Anatomy

Because these lines are often related to repeated flexion of the obese neck, they frequently cannot be softened or removed with BoNT-A injection. However, some of these lines may be caused by attachments of the SMAS within the neck, which represents an appropriate target for BoNT-A treatment.

Technique

The injection technique is similar to that described for vertical platysmal bands, but the injections are often given in the deep intradermal plane along the lines, using an interrupted technique. A total of 10 to 15 U is injected.

Follow-up

If inadequate correction of the horizontal platysmal bands is noted, additional BoNT-A may be injected a minimum of 7 days after the initial injections, at which time the expected effect of the initial BoNT-A should be achieved. However, BoNT-A's failure to smooth the lines likely indicates that the lines are not the result of insertion of the SMAS.

Complications

The same complications described in the vertical platysmal bands section apply to injections for horizontal platysmal bands.

9.4 Conclusion

The use of BoNT for the reduction of hyperfunctional facial lines is a commonly performed nonsurgical facial rejuvenation procedure because of the remarkable safety, reliability, and patient satisfaction associated with its use over the past decade. Current trends in facial rejuvenation are characterized by decreased treatment doses that modulate the activity rather than paralyze the muscles of facial expression. There is also increasing use of adjunctive procedures, including volume augmentation and skin resurfacing in conjunction with BoNT treatment. The future of facial aesthetic medicine and surgery will undoubtedly bring new formulations of BoNT, as well as new, minimally invasive procedures into the clinician's armamentarium. However, safe and effective administration of BoNT will always depend on a thorough understanding of the muscular and vascular anatomy of the face and neck, as well as proper patient counseling regarding the anticipated aesthetic outcome.

9.5 Key Points/Pearls

- Botulinum neurotoxin is a safe and effective temporary treatment of hyperfunctional facial lines.
- OnabotulinumtoxinA (Botox, Allergan plc, Irvine, CA) is FDA-approved for the treatment of moderate to severe glabellar lines, moderate to severe lateral canthal lines/periocular lines, and moderate to severe forehead lines associated with frontalis muscle activity.
- AbobotulinumtoxinA (Dysport; Ipsen Biopharmaceuticals Inc, Basking Ridge, NJ) and incobotulinumtoxinA (Xeomin; Merz Pharmaceuticals, Greensboro, NC) are currently approved only for the temporary treatment of moderate to severe glabellar lines.

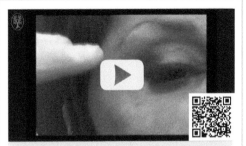

Video 9.1 Cosmetic: crow's feet. The patient is asked to squint so that the areas of maximum line formation may be seen. Then, three injections of toxin (2.5 U/0.1 mL) along the orbital rim at least 1 cm from the lateral rectus attachment. [0:58]

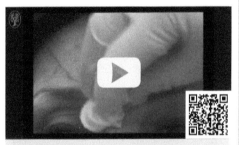

Video 9.2 Cosmetic: frown lines. You see in this video a "Blitzer" safety triangle drawn. If you place one point between the medial portion of the brows and then another at 1 cm above the superior orbital rim at the mid papillary line bilaterally, a triangle can be drawn. Anything within this triangle is safe to inject. Leaving a bit of lateral frontalis muscle allows for some mimetic action and expressivity. You see in this video the corrugator muscle being injected within the triangle to eliminate frown lines. Injection of 2.5 U/0.1 mL is given in five places. [0:52]

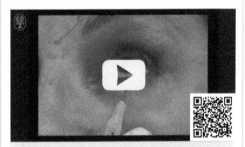

Video 9.3 Cosmetic: lower eyelid. These injections are given just subcutaneously along the tarsal plate. They should not be given medial to the midpupillary line to prevent weakening of the pumping action of the lower lid and producing epiphora. These injections will reduce the lower lid lines and make the lid opening rounder. Injections are 1.0 U/0.05 mL in two places along the lower lid. [0:32]

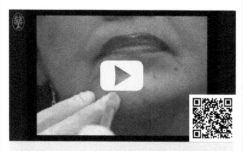

Video 9.4 Cosmetic: mentalis. These injections treat the "peau d'orange" skin changes. Each mentalis muscle is injected with 2.5 to 5 U/0.1 mL. The injections should be given no higher than halfway superior from the inferior border of mandible to the upper border of the lower lip. Above this line threatens to weaken the orbicularis oris and may produce drooling or dysarthria. [0:52]

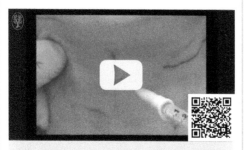

Video 9.5 Cosmetic: platysma. The anterior edge and posterior edge of the platysma muscles are marked. A "ladder" of horizontal lines is drawn about 2 cm apart. Using an EMG needle, the ladder lines are skewered observing for good muscle EMG activity and 2.5 U/0.1 mL is injected in each pass as the needle is removed. For large anterior bands, the band can be grasped between fingers and extra toxin injected into the bands. [2:14]

References

[1] Carruthers JA, Lowe NJ, Menter MA, et al. BOTOX Glabellar Lines I Study Group. A multicenter, double-blind, randomized, placebo-controlled study of the efficacy and safety of botulinum toxin type A in the treatment of glabellar lines. J Am Acad Dermatol.; 46(6):840–849

[2] Lowe NJ, Lask G, Yamauchi P, Moore D. Bilateral, double-blind, randomized comparison of 3 doses of botulinum toxin type A and placebo in patients with crow's feet. J Am Acad Dermatol.; 47(6):834–840

[3] American Society for Aesthetic Plastic Surgery. Cosmetic surgery national data bank: 2017 statistics. Available at: www.surgery.org/media/statistics. Accessed July 10, 2019

[4] Carruthers JDA, Glogau RG, Blitzer A, Facial Aesthetics Consensus Group Faculty. Advances in facial rejuvenation: botulinum toxin type a, hyaluronic acid dermal fillers, and combination therapies–consensus recommendations. Plast Reconstr Surg.; 121(5) Suppl:5S–30S, quiz 31S–36S

[5] Sattler G. Current and future botulinum neurotoxin type A preparations in aesthetics: a literature review. J Drugs Dermatol.; 9(9):1065–1071

[6] Kane M, Donofrio L, Ascher B, et al. Expanding the use of neurotoxins in facial aesthetics: a consensus panel's assessment and recommendations. J Drugs Dermatol.; 9(1) Suppl:s7–s22, quiz s23–s25

[7] Ascher B, Talarico S, Cassuto D, et al. International consensus recommendations on the aesthetic usage of botulinum toxin type A (Speywood Unit)–Part II: wrinkles on the middle and lower face, neck and chest. J Eur Acad Dermatol Venereol.; 24 (11):1285–1295

[8] Carruthers A, Carruthers J, Lei X, Pogoda JM, Eadie N, Brin MF. OnabotulinumtoxinA treatment of mild glabellar lines in repose. Dermatol Surg.; 36 Suppl 4:2168–2171

[9] Lee SH, Min HJ, Kim YW, Cheon YW. The efficacy and safety of early postoperative botulinum toxin A injection for facial scars. Aesthetic Plast Surg.; 42(2):530–537

[10] Wynn R, Bentsianov BL, Blitzer A. Botulinum toxin injection for the lower face and neck. Oper Tech Otol Head Neck Surg.; 15:139–142

[11] Baumann L, Martin LK. Myobloc for facial wrinkles. Oper Tech Otol Head Neck Surg.; 15:143–146

[12] Cliff SH, Judodihardjo H, Eltringham E. Different formulations of botulinum toxin type A have different migration characteristics: a double-blind, randomized study. J Cosmet Dermatol.; 7(1):50–54

[13] Cheng CM. Cosmetic use of botulinum toxin type A in the elderly. Clin Interv Aging.; 2(1):81–83

[14] Li Y, Dong W, Wang M, Xu N. Investigation of the efficacy and safety of topical vibration anesthesia to reduce pain from cosmetic botulinum toxin a injections in Chinese patients: a multicenter, randomized, self-controlled study. Dermatol Surg.

[15] Borodic G. Immunologic resistance after repeated botulinum toxin type a injections for facial rhytides. Ophthal Plast Reconstr Surg.; 22(3):239–240

[16] Lowe NJ. Cosmetic therapy: glabellar and forehead area. Oper Tech Otol Head Neck Surg.; 15:128–133

[17] Carruthers J, Carruthers A. Aesthetic uses of botulinum toxin A in the periocular region and mid and lower face. Oper Tech Otol Head Neck Surg.; 15(2):134–138

[18] Polo M. Botulinum toxin type A in the treatment of excessive gingival display. Am J Orthod Dentofacial Orthop.; 127(2):214–218, quiz 261

10
Botulinum Neurotoxin for Upper and Lower Esophageal Spasm

Nwanmegha Young and Brian E. Benson

Summary

The upper and lower esophageal sphincters play critical roles in the regulation of the passage of liquids and solids. Hyperfunctioning of the muscles within sphincters can lead to dysfunction manifesting clinically as dysphagia. Injection of botulinum toxin into these muscles can reduce the hyperfunctioning and relieve the dysphagia. For the upper esophageal sphincter, the injections can be given percutaneously or endoscopically. The lower esophageal sphincter injections are typically done endoscopically. Studies have shown that these injections are safe with minimal complications.

Keywords: achalasia, dysphagia, upper esophageal sphincter, cricopharyngeus muscle, lower esophageal sphincter, cardiospasm

10.1 Introduction

Dysphagia, or impaired swallowing ability, is a very common disorder that can have adverse effects on quality of life and overall health. Although over 20% of the adult population experiences dysphagia several times a month,[1] the impact on overall health and quality of life can range from minimal, in the case of mild dysphagia, to life threatening, in the case of severe dysphagia. Dysphagia may result from dysfunction of any of the components involved in the complex neuromuscular interaction that facilitates the swallowing mechanism. While there are three functional categorizations of dysphagia (oral, oropharyngeal, esophageal), the only two types that respond favorably to botulinum neurotoxin (BoNT) injection are *oropharyngeal*, which refers to difficulty in the passage of a food bolus from the oropharynx into the esophagus, and *esophageal*, which refers to disturbances of the passage of the food bolus within the esophagus itself.[2] Hyperfunction of any of the muscles involved in swallowing is a frequent cause of dysphagia, although in most cases of moderate or severe dysphagia, there are multiple, significant deficits related to muscle strength, coordination, and sensation. With regard to isolated hyperfunctional dysphagia, failure of relaxation of the cricopharyngeus (CP) muscle is the most common cause of oropharyngeal dysphagia, and hypertonicity of the lower sphincter is associated with esophageal dyshagia.[3,4]

Treatment of these disorders depends on the etiology of the dysphagia (stroke, neurodegenerative disease, congenital disorders, high vagal lesions, postlaryngectomy, etc.), and may include surgery, medications, or swallowing therapy, or some combination of them. When the main cause of dysphagia is hyperfunctional muscles, chemodenervation with BoNT is a reasonable treatment option. This chapter reviews the anatomy, physiology, and management of hyperfunctional swallowing disorders that may affect the pharyngoesophageal phase of swallowing.

10.2 Anatomy and Physiology

The esophagus forms a muscular conduit that connects the hypopharynx to the stomach. It is approximately 18 to 26 cm in length and topographically is divided into three regions: cervical, esophageal, and abdominal. The upper or cervical segment is composed of striated muscle, whereas the lower or abdominal part is composed of smooth muscle. The esophageal region is a mixed transition zone composed of both muscle types. The upper esophageal sphincter (UES) and lower esophageal sphincter (LES), in conjunction with the esophagus, are responsible for anterograde transport of nutrients and for preventing the retrograde transport of gastric contents. Hypertonicity, that is, decreased or absent relaxation, in these zones, leads to dysphagia.

10.2.1 Anatomy and Physiology of the Upper Esophageal Sphincter

At each end of the esophagus, there lie high-pressure zones.[5,6] The UES is a 2- to 4-cm high-pressure zone at the junction of the hypopharynx and the esophagus (▶ Fig. 10.1, ▶ Fig. 10.2).

The most prominent component of the UES is the CP muscle, which constitutes the lower third of the UES. The upper two-thirds of the UES comprise the lower portion of the inferior pharyngeal constrictor. The fibers of the CP muscle originate and insert in the dorsolateral aspect of the cricoid cartilage, which defines the anterior aspect of the UES. Although the innervation of the CP muscle remains a matter of debate, the most prominent contributions are from the vagus and glossopharyngeal nerves as well as the sympathetic nerve fibers.[7,8,9] Innervation of the CP muscle is ipsilateral; therefore, the two halves of the CP muscle function independently. Acetylcholine is the primary neurotransmitter, thereby making the UES an attractive target for BoNT therapy in cases of hypertonicity. The CP is unique among the muscles of the neck, in that it maintains a high intraluminal pressure during respiration and speech, relaxing only during deglutition.

10.2.2 Anatomy and Physiology of the Lower Esophageal Sphincter

The LES, also referred to as the gastroesophageal sphincter, cardiac sphincter, or esophageal sphincter, is located at the junction of the esophagus and the stomach. It has intrinsic (esophageal) and extrinsic (diaphragmatic) components (▶ Fig. 10.3).

Lower esophageal spasm, or achalasia, is a primary esophageal motility disorder characterized by failure of a hypertensive LES to relax coupled with the absence of esophageal peristalsis. These abnormalities cause a functional obstruction at the gastroesophageal junction, leading to esophageal dysphagia, regurgitation, and weight loss. LES pressure and relaxation are regulated by excitatory (e.g., acetylcholine, substance P) and inhibitory (e.g., nitric oxide, vasoactive intestinal peptide) neurotransmitters. Patients with LES achalasia lack nonadrenergic, noncholinergic, inhibitory ganglion cells, causing an imbalance in excitatory and inhibitory neurotransmission.[3,4] The result is a hypertensive nonrelaxed esophageal sphincter.

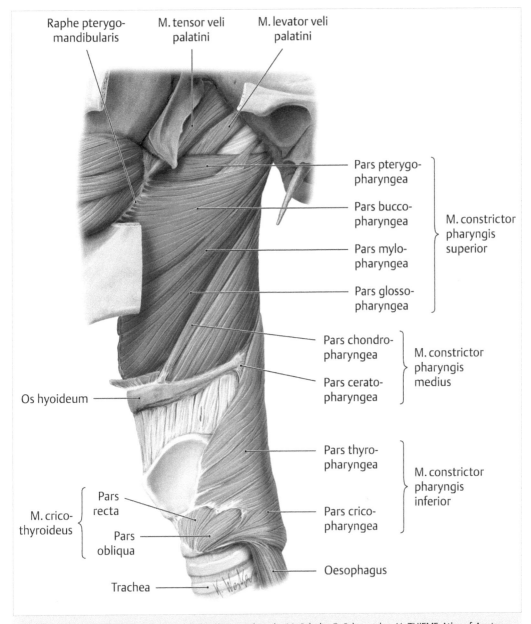

Fig. 10.1 Upper esophageal sphincter muscles. (From Schuenke M, Schulte E, Schumacher U. THIEME Atlas of Anatomy: Head, Neck, and Neuroanatomy. Illustrations by Voll M and Wesker K. 2nd Ed. New York: Thieme Medical Publishers; 2016.)

10.3 Dysfunction of the Upper Esophageal Sphincter

Failure of the UES to relax, termed cricopharyngeal achalasia (CA), can cause severe dysphagia. CA is a characteristic symptom in a variety of neurologic disorders including lesions of the skull base and stroke. UES hypertonicity is also associated with distal esophageal reflux[10]; so in mildly symptomatic patients, treatment with proton pump inhibitors may be effective. Clinical symptoms of CA include globus sensation and dysphagia. In newborns, an esophagram confirms the diagnosis. In adults, however, the diagnosis

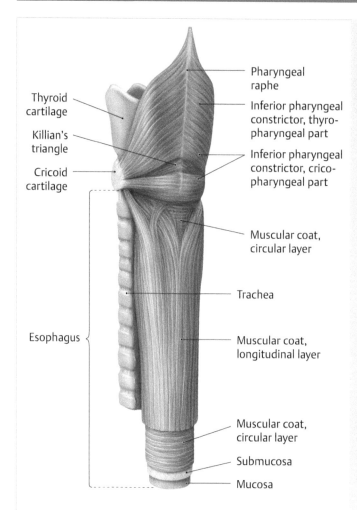

Thyroid cartilage

Killian's triangle

Cricoid cartilage

Esophagus

Pharyngeal raphe

Inferior pharyngeal constrictor, thyro-pharyngeal part

Inferior pharyngeal constrictor, crico-pharyngeal part

Muscular coat, circular layer

Trachea

Muscular coat, longitudinal layer

Muscular coat, circular layer

Submucosa

Mucosa

Fig. 10.2 Esophageal wall, oblique left posterior view. (From Schuenke M, Schulte E, Schumacher U. THIEME Atlas of Anatomy: Head, Neck, and Neuroanatomy. Illustrations by Voll M and Wesker K. 2nd Ed. New York: Thieme Medical Publishers; 2016.)

is best aided by manometry or electromyography (EMG). However, equivocal or negative findings with these testing modalities, which have significant technical aspects, do not rule out CA.

CA can be managed with a variety of treatments, including mechanical dilatation, BoNT injection, and CP myotomy. The definitive treatment of CA remains CP myotomy, via either an endoscopic or open transcervical approach.[11] Injection of BoNT into the CP muscle, either percutaneously or endoscopically under general anesthesia, has shown benefit in 70 to 100% of patients in noncontrolled series.[12] The effects of the injection lasted

between 4 months and 1 year. Therefore, BoNT injection is not only an attractive nonsurgical alternative treatment for CA but also a useful tool to identify which patients could be expected to experience benefit from CP myotomy. An important exception is patients with fibrosis of the CP, who will not experience benefit from BoNT, but may benefit from dilation or myotomy. Ahsan et al[13] reported a series of five patients with CA and severe dysphagia. Prior to treatment, all patients were dependent on feeding tubes. After BoNT injection, all patients had improvement of their swallowing and four out of five patients were able to have their

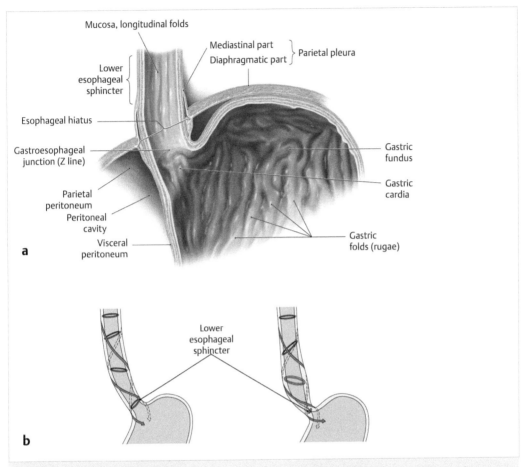

Fig. 10.3 (a,b) Lower esophageal sphincter. (From Schuenke M, Schulte E, Schumacher U. THIEME Atlas of Anatomy: Head, Neck, and Neuroanatomy. Illustrations by Voll M and Wesker K. 2nd Ed. New York: Thieme Medical Publishers; 2016.)

feeding tubes removed. Murry et al[14] showed in a series of 13 patients that BoNT injection of the CP in the office improved swallow safety and reduced the need for nonoral feeding. In laryngectomized patients, Lightbody et al[15] showed that BoNT injection into the pharyngoesophageal segment is effective in treating dysphagia, dysphonia, and tracheoesophageal prosthesis valve leak.

10.3.1 Alternative Treatments

Large bore bougie dilation under general anesthesia[16] and transnasal unsedated balloon dilation[17] are effective and safe alternatives to BoNT for patients in whom BoNT is contraindicated. The advantage of unsedated balloon dilation of the UES is that there is no risk of airway compromise and migration of the toxin. The effect of the dilation lasts for approximately the same time as BoNT in most patients.

10.4 Dysfunction of the Lower Esophageal Sphincter

Lower esophageal sphincter (LES) spasm, referred to as achalasia, esophageal achalasia, and cardiospasm, is a primary esophageal motility disorder characterized by failure of a hypertensive LES to relax and the absence of esophageal peristalsis. These abnormalities cause a functional obstruction at the gastroesophageal junction, leading to dysphagia, regurgitation, weight loss, and occasionally chest pain. These symptoms may also be mimicked by neoplasm and infection (Chagas disease). Treatments for achalasia include medications, balloon dilation, and myotomy. Calcium channel blockers and nitrates have shown short-term efficacy, but their use is limited by side effects, including headache, dizziness, hypotension, and peripheral edema.[18] Although the durability of response in patients undergoing myotomy or balloon dilation techniques is superior than that in patients who undergo BoNT injection, intrasphincteric injection of BoNT has been demonstrated to be an extremely safe and effective treatment for those patients who are not good surgical candidates, or who prefer to avoid surgical risks.[19]

10.5 Workup

Evaluation of dysphagia requires a thorough history and physical examination, often including fiberoptic evaluation of the oropharynx, endolarynx, and hypopharynx, and of the esophagus and stomach. Additional studies are as follows:

- Radiologic studies:
  - Modified barium swallow.
  - Barium esophagram.
- Functional evaluation:
  - Flexible fiberoptic evaluation of swallowing (with or without) sensory testing.
  - Manometry.
- Nerve studies:
  - Electromyography.

10.5.1 Upper Esophageal Sphincter Workup

The radiographic hallmark of CP achalasia, the "cricopharyngeal bar," represents the protrusion of the CP muscle into the digestive tract as the bolus of radiopaque material passes through the UES. However, the absence of a CP bar does not rule out the possibility of UES hyperfunction if the history and physical examination findings are suggestive (▶ Fig. 10.4). Fiberoptic pharyngoscopy may reveal pooling of secretions with the pyriform sinus region on the affected side. EMG studies may reveal the lack of cessation of electrical activity, although a decrease in signal is usually noted during swallowing, even in patients with CP achalasia.

10.5.2 Lower Esophageal Sphincter Workup

Esophageal manometry frequently reveals high resting LES pressure, incomplete relaxation of the LES during swallowing, and absent of esophageal peristalsis. A barium esophagram shows a proximal dilated esophagus. The distal esophagus is narrowed and classically described as resembling a bird's beak.

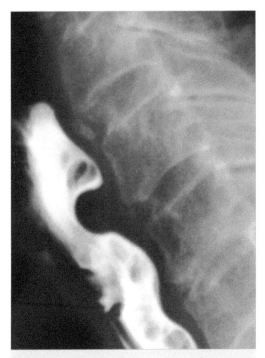

Fig. 10.4 Cricopharyngeal bar.

10.6 Upper Esophageal Sphincter Technique

10.6.1 Percutaneous

The patient is placed in the supine position. The surgeon stands at the side of the patient and rotates the larynx with one hand while using the contralateral hand to pass a Teflon-coated hollow EMG recording needle through the skin and into the CP muscle. Entry into the CP muscle is confirmed by the EMG's demonstrating activity during rest and relaxation during swallowing, even in hyperkinetic states. The effective amount injected is usually 10 to 20 units (U) on each side.

10.6.2 Post-Laryngectomy

In patients who have undergone total laryngectomy, cricopharyngeal dysfunction, or pharyngoesophageal spasm, commonly results in dysphagia and TEP malfunction, even if cricopharyngeal myotomy has been performed at the time of the laryngectomy. Diagnostic and therapeutic utility of EMG is extremely limited, due to postoperative and postradiation fibrosis. While fluoroscopic guidance has been described, the authors have found high-dose (50–100 U) injection technique of the suprastomal region. Care is taken to withdraw the plunger to avoid inadvertent intravascular or intraluminal injection. Preinjection workup must include evaluation for pharyngoesophageal stricture or recurrence of neoplasm.

10.6.3 Endoscopic

Under general anesthesia, a rigid endoscope is positioned in the postcricoid region and placed in suspension. A bivalved hypopharyngoscope, with sufficient length to expose the UES, is optimal for visualization, although sometimes a laryngoscope or esophagoscope can provide adequate visualization. Because the cricoid cartilage is pushed anteriorly with the positioning of the scope, the cricopharyngeal muscle comes into view as a posterior bulky crescent at the cricopharyngeal inlet. This is similar to the placement of a laryngoscope for repair of a Zenker diverticulum. A blunt tip probe is used to palpate the horizontally oriented muscle to confirm that the correct area is exposed. If the scope is not placed deeply enough, the inferior constrictor muscle may be inadvertently injected instead of the CP, and this would produce a worsening of the patient's dysphagia.

Once the cricopharyngeal muscle is verified, it is injected under direct visualization. Laryngeal injection needles can be used or, alternatively, a butterfly needle with its wings cut off can be used to deliver the toxin. Typically, one or two areas of the muscle are injected with BoNT on each side of the posterior portion of the muscle in the 5 o'clock and 7 o'clock positions. The anterior aspect of the muscle should not be injected, as this may cause stridor due to paralysis of the posterior cricoarytenoid muscle. The amount injected varies widely between authors, from 5 to 100 U, with typical doses used by the authors ranging from 15 to 40 U.

An advantage of performing this procedure under general anesthesia is the opportunity to additionally carry out rigid cervical esophagoscopy to rule out causes of dysphagia other than CA. Some practitioners will also perform bougie dilation of the CP prior to injecting BoNT.

10.6.4 Complications and Pitfalls

For the transcutaneous approach, adequate laryngeal rotation for injection may not be achieved in all patients. This technique is moderately difficult, especially in older patients who may have neck rigidity, kyphosis, and/or a low-laying larynx. Diffusion of the toxin to the posterior cricoarytenoid muscles can cause a bilateral vocal cord paresis. If severe enough, it can require a temporary tracheostomy. Migration of the toxin into the pharyngeal constrictors can worsen dysphagia symptoms so that a temporary feeding tube may be required. For these reasons, we recommend low-dose injections, staged left and right injections when the percutaneous technique is used, and a low threshold to offer alternative treatment modalities. Special care should also be exercised in patients whose esophagram or manometry study shows retrograde peristaltic waves, as increased reflux and regurgitation will likely occur if the CP muscle is weakened.

10.7 Lower Esophageal Sphincter Technique

10.7.1 Endoscopic

This technique can be done with either rigid or flexible esophagoscopes in an outpatient setting. The position of the LES is identified by visualization of the Z-line and the typical narrow segment of the cardia region. Twenty units of BoNT are then injected into four quadrants (total of 80 U). No postinjection radiographic imaging is required. The patients can begin eating 2 hours after the procedure.

10.7.2 Complications and Pitfalls

The rate of serious complications is extremely low. Twenty percent of patients may develop chest discomfort after the procedure, and 10% may develop gastroesophageal reflux.[20]

10.8 Follow-up

The injection may be repeated if symptoms return.

10.9 Conclusion

Botulinum neurotoxin injection into the various hyperfunctioning muscle groups of the hypopharynx and esophagus can be a safe and effective means of temporarily relieving the associated dysphagia symptoms. If the BoNT treatment proves effective, then it can be repeated every 4 months, or as needed. Use of BoNT also plays a very important role as a diagnostic modality to identify patients who will benefit from surgical myotomy.

10.10 Key Points/Pearls

- The cricopharyngeal muscle is the most important contributor to the upper esophageal sphincter and is the target for botulinum toxin.
- The cricopharyngeal muscle can be injected either endoscopically or percutaneously.
- Care must be taken to not allow diffusion of botulinum toxin into the posterior cricoarytenoid muscles.
- Lower esophageal sphincter is injected endoscopically in four quadrants.
- The rate of complications is extremely low.

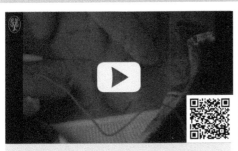

Video 10.1 Cricopharyngeus muscle. These injections are given bilaterally into the cricopharyngeus muscle. A dose of 2.5 U/0.1 mL is given at two sites on each side of the pharynx. These injections should be given 1 cm below the bottom of the cricoid cartilage. The needle is advanced until activity is heard. If in the cricopharyngeus muscle, the activity should abate on swallowing. [2:03]

References

[1] Wilkins T, Gillies RA, Thomas AM, Wagner PJ. The prevalence of dysphagia in primary care patients: a HamesNet Research Network study. J Am Board Fam Med.; 20(2):144–150

[2] Spieker MR. Evaluating dysphagia. Am Fam Physician.; 61 (12):3639–3648

[3] Annese V, Bassotti G. Non-surgical treatment of esophageal achalasia. World J Gastroenterol.; 12(36):5763–5766

[4] D'Onofrio V, Miletto P, Leandro G, Iaquinto G. Long-term follow-up of achalasia patients treated with botulinum toxin. Dig Liver Dis.; 34(2):105–110

[5] Pandolfino JE, Fox MR, Bredenoord AJ, Kahrilas PJ. High-resolution manometry in clinical practice: utilizing pressure topography to classify oesophageal motility abnormalities. Neurogastroenterol Motil.; 21(8):796–806– Review

[6] Kahrilas PJ, Ghosh SK, Pandolfino JE. Esophageal motility disorders in terms of pressure topography: the Chicago Classification. J Clin Gastroenterol.; 42(5):627–635

[7] Mu L, Sanders I. The innervation of the human upper esophageal sphincter. Dysphagia.; 11(4):234–238

[8] Mu L, Sanders I. Neuromuscular organization of the human upper esophageal sphincter. Ann Otol Rhinol Laryngol.; 107 (5, Pt 1):370–377

[9] Sasaki CT, Kim YH, Sims HS, Czibulka A. Motor innervation of the human cricopharyngeus muscle. Ann Otol Rhinol Laryngol.; 108(12):1132–1139

[10] Tokashiki R, Funato N, Suzuki M. Globus sensation and increased upper esophageal sphincter pressure with distal esophageal acid perfusion. Eur Arch Otorhinolaryngol.; 267 (5):737–741

[11] Pitman M, Weissbrod P. Endoscopic CO2 laser cricopharyngeal myotomy. Laryngoscope.; 119(1):45–53

[12] Blitzer A, Brin MF. Use of botulinum toxin for diagnosis and management of cricopharyngeal achalasia. Otolaryngol Head Neck Surg.; 116(3):328–330

[13] Ahsan SF, Meleca RJ, Dworkin JP. Botulinum toxin injection of the cricopharyngeus muscle for the treatment of dysphagia. Otolaryngol Head Neck Surg.; 122(5):691–695

[14] Murry T, Wasserman T, Carrau RL, Castillo B. Injection of botulinum toxin A for the treatment of dysfunction of the upper esophageal sphincter. Am J Otolaryngol.; 26(3):157–162

[15] Lightbody KA, Wilkie MD, Kinshuck AJ, et al. Injection of botulinum toxin for the treatment of post-laryngectomy pharyngoesophageal spasm-related disorders. Ann R Coll Surg Engl.; 97(7):508–512

[16] Clary MS, Daniero JJ, Keith SW, Boon MS, Spiegel JR. Efficacy of large-diameter dilatation in cricopharyngeal dysfunction. Laryngoscope.; 121(12):2521–2525

[17] Rees CJ, Fordham T, Belafsky PC. Transnasal balloon dilation of the esophagus. Arch Otolaryngol Head Neck Surg.; 135(8): 781–783

[18] Moawad FJ, Wong RKh. Modern management of achalasia. Curr Opin Gastroenterol.; 26(4):384–388

[19] Wang L, Li YM, Li L. Meta-analysis of randomized and controlled treatment trials for achalasia. Dig Dis Sci.; 54(11): 2303–2311

[20] Walzer N, Hirano I. Achalasia. Gastroenterol Clin North Am.; 37(4):807–825, viii

11
Botulinum Neurotoxin for Palatal Myoclonus

Ajay E. Chitkara, Catherine F. Sinclair, and Daniel Novakovic

Summary

Palatal myoclonus (PM) is a movement disorder affecting the soft palate muscles. It can be classified into essential palatal tremor or symptomatic palatal tremor. PM can present with symptoms of clicking tinnitus or perceived palatal movements. Botulinum toxin injections directed at the tensor veli palatini and/or levator veli palatini muscles can assist with symptomatic control.

Keywords: palatal myoclonus, palatal tremor, botulinum toxin, movement disorder, soft palate, tensor veli palatini, levator veli palatini

11.1 Introduction

Palatal myoclonus (PM) is a movement disorder characterized by involuntary rhythmic muscular contraction of the soft palate. It was categorized as palatal tremor (PT) at the First International Congress of Movement Disorders in 1990, though the terms are often used interchangeably in the literature.[1] PT is subclassified into symptomatic palatal tremor (SPT) and essential palatal tremor (EPT). SPT is typically one facet of a constellation of symptoms involving the head, neck, and face. SPT is infrequently symptomatic at the level of the palate (8% of cases), and rarely requires medical treatment. By contrast, EPT is frequently symptomatic and usually generates a symptomatic ear clicking tinnitus secondary to involuntary palate contractions. This clicking may be audible to others. Additional symptoms include nonaudible awareness of palatal movements and rhinolalia.[2] The end-organ difference between SPT and EPT is thought to be the reason for the variance of symptoms: SPT is posited to involve the levator veli palatini (LVP; cranial nerves IX and X), whereas EPT is presumed to involve the tensor veli palatini (TVP; cranial nerve V) (▶ Fig. 11.1, ▶ Table 11.1).

Contraction of the tensor is associated with the rapid opening of the eustachian tube, creating a sudden drop in tubal surface tension resulting in the often-described audible snap, crack, or pop (▶ Fig. 11.2).[3] PT may involve one or both sides of the soft palate, oscillating at a frequency of 0.5 to 300 Hz. The typical age for EPT is 25 to 35 years compared with 45 years for patients with SPT, with an equal male-to-female incidence.[1,2,4] Despite the subclassification of PT into SPT and EPT, there is evidence supporting a spectrum of PT disorders, as some patients do not clearly fit into one subclass or the other.[1]

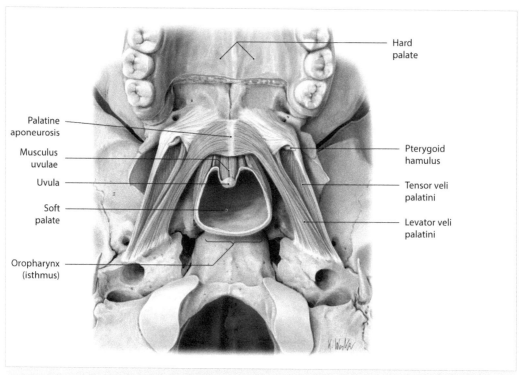

Fig. 11.1 Muscles of the soft palate. (From Schuenke M, Schulte E, Schumacher U. THIEME Atlas of Anatomy: Head, Neck, and Neuroanatomy. Illustrations by Voll M and Wesker K. 2nd Ed. New York: Thieme Medical Publishers; 2016.)

Table 11.1 Muscles of the soft palate

Muscle	Origin	Insertion	Innervation	Action
Tensor veli palatini	Medial pterygoid plate (scaphoid fossa); sphenoid bone (spine); cartilage of pharyngotympanic tube	Palatine aponeurosis	Medial pterygoid n. (cranial nerve V_3 via otic ganglion)	Tightens soft palate; opens inlet to pharyngotympanic tube (during swallowing, yawning)
Levator veli palatini	Cartilage of pharyngotympanic tube; temporal bone (petrous part)			Raises soft palate to horizontal position
Musculus uvulae	Uvula (mucosa)	Palatine aponeurosis; posterior nasal spine	Accessory n. (cranial nerve XI, cranial part) via pharyngeal plexus	Shortens and raises uvula
Palatoglossus	Tongue (side)	Palatine aponeurosis	(vagus n., cranial nerve X)	Elevates tongue (posterior position); pulls soft palate onto tongue
Palatopharyngeus				Tightens soft palate; during swallowing pulls pharyngeal walls superiorly, anteriorly, and medially

Source: Adapted with permission from Gilroy AM, MacPherson BR, Ross LM. Atlas of Anatomy. New York, NY: Thieme; 2008:545.

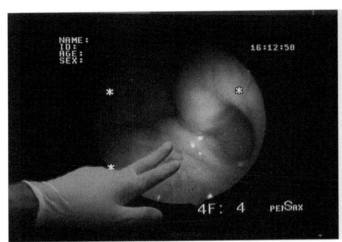

Fig. 11.2 Eustachian tube orifice.

11.2 Workup

The diagnosis of PM relies on disease history and a neuro-otorhinolaryngologic evaluation. The most common complaint is the characteristic clicking tinnitus, which may be audible to the examiner. In essential PT (which more commonly presents with palatal symptoms), imaging and laboratory evaluations are usually normal. Despite the paucity of diagnostic findings, neurologic assessment is often indicated to define or exclude any associated or underlying abnormality. Symptomatic PT is usually devoid of any palate-specific symptoms, though it is associated with other neurologic movement disorders of the head and neck which may include the larynx, pharynx, face, or other structures controlled by the brainstem or cerebellum. SPT often presents with other clinical findings including dysarthria, nystagmus, and ataxia[1] and is often synchronous with the extrapalatal myoclonic structures.[4] Symptomatic PT warrants a full neurologic evaluation.

The most common form of SPT is secondary to a structural lesion of the brainstem or cerebellum with palatal symptoms developing at a median of 10 months after the injury and persisting throughout life. Hypertrophic olivary degeneration is typically identified on magnetic resonance imaging with increased signal intensity and enlargement of the inferior olive or dentato-olivary tract on T2-weighted/fluid-attenuated inversion recovery and proton-weighted images.[5] SPT has been associated with numerous systemic metabolic, immunologic, infectious, and traumatic disorders. Causes of SPT include the following:

- Hereditary syndrome.
- Familial leukodystrophy.
- Neurodegenerative disorders.
- Vascular: hemorrhagic or ischemic cerebral insult.
- Trauma.
- Viral encephalitis.
- Malaria.
- Multiple sclerosis.
- Cerebrotendinous xanthomatosis.
- Behçet disease.
- Krabbe disease.
- Sclerosing leukoencephalopathy.
- Immunologic.
- Brainstem tumors or surgery.
- Drug induced.

The potential etiology of EPT is heterogenous with theories supporting the presence of a central mechanism generating the abnormal movement. Local mechanical and inflammatory causes have also been postulated with 40% reporting that myoclonic symptoms began after viral upper respiratory tract infection.[2] Some patients can voluntarily elicit the movement and there are a significant number of cases with psychogenic origin.[1,6]

11.3 Treatment and Technique

Management of PM with botulinum neurotoxin (BoNT) has been shown to be an effective treatment with minimal side effects. Chemodenervation injections are targeted either laterally toward the TVP or medially toward the LVP depending on the primary presenting symptom. Regardless of the underlying subclassification of PT, treatment is primarily targeted toward the predominant symptom(s). Thus, treatment should initially target the tensor muscle when the goal of therapy is to remediate the clicking tinnitus. Conversely, when perceived palatal movements are the predominant symptom, treatment should initially target the levator muscle.[2] In the United States, onabotulinumtoxinA is the most widely used formulation of BoNT-A. Typical treatment consists of one or two injection sites per side of the soft palate, placing 2.5 units (U) per injection site for an initial dose of 2.5 to 5 U per side. Reported dose ranges can vary from 2.5 to 15 U of BoNT-A per side of the palate.[7,8,9,10] These injections are best performed under electromyographic guidance with a 27-gauge monopolar injection needle to maximize precision in locating the target muscle. The BoNT is diluted to 2.5 U per 0.1 mL of saline (4 mL saline per 100 U vial of onabotulinumtoxinA), with a starting dose of 2.5 to 5 U to each muscle target. Where higher doses are required, a more concentrated dilution of 5 U per 0.1 mL saline is utilized in order to minimize excessive diffusion to surrounding local musculature. Injections are typically performed in the ambulatory setting with the patient seated in a treatment chair. Topical anesthesia may be applied to the pharynx. Under direct transoral visualization, the injection needle is placed approximately 3 to 5 mm posterior to the posterior edge of the hard palate. Medial injections are performed on either side of the uvula into the LVP. Injections lateral to the hamulus will target the LVP (▶ Fig. 11.3, ▶ Fig. 11.4). One or both sites can be treated in the same setting, although we recommend staging the injections by 2 weeks to minimize the risk of side effects.

Placement of the injection too far posterior or anterior in the soft palate may result in dysphagia due to chemodenervation of the posterior or anterior fasciculus of the palatopharyngeus muscles, respectively, with limited improvement in the clicking tinnitus. The patient returns for follow-up 2 to 4 weeks after the initial injection, at which time the symptomatic benefit and any untoward effects can be assessed. A booster injection may be required at the follow-up if the patient is not realizing adequate benefit from the initial injection dose. The dose at follow-up, and at subsequent visits, should be titrated according to the patient's response to the prior injections. After the first one to three injection cycles, most patients can limit their follow-up to the injection visits only. At each visit, the treatment outcome is reviewed with the patient. When necessary, adjustments are made in the dosing and occasionally the location of injection sites to maximize symptom improvement and minimize the downside of the injections. Using the aforementioned regime, symptomatic improvement has been reported in 85.7% of patients with EPT. Occasionally, injections into the TVP do not adequately extinguish the tremor. Some clinicians have had success injecting the LVP or injecting the salpingopharyngeus

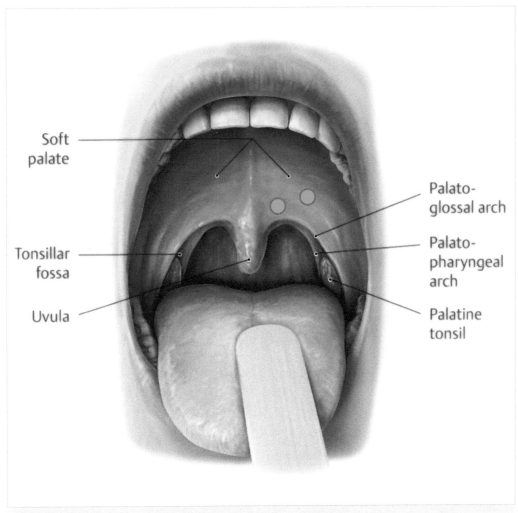

Soft palate

Tonsillar fossa

Uvula

Palato-glossal arch

Palato-pharyngeal arch

Palatine tonsil

Fig. 11.3 Injection points on palate. (From Schuenke M, Schulte E, Schumacher U. THIEME Atlas of Anatomy: Head, Neck, and Neuroanatomy. Illustrations by Voll M and Wesker K. 2nd Ed. New York: Thieme Medical Publishers; 2016.)

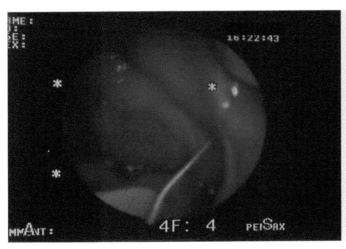

Fig. 11.4 Palate injection.

muscle via an endoscopic endonasal approach.[11,12]

Most patients require repeated injections at 3- to 6-month intervals. Though the duration of effect of the BoNT is approximately 4 months, some patients have reported resolution of symptoms after a single injection cycle. It is thought that some of these patients may have demonstrated a psychogenic variant of PM.[13,14] Pharmacologic management of PM may be attempted, though it is rarely successful as the sole treatment. In patients who are treated with systemic medication, BoNT injections may provide complementary benefit to the PM.

11.4 Complications and Pitfalls

Patients undergoing BoNT therapy are counseled regarding the general risks associated with use of the toxin. The typical dose range used for PM is a relatively low total systemic dose, and therefore poses an extremely low risk of systemic side effects.

Most adverse outcomes relate to inadvertent paralysis of the local musculature involved in moving the soft palate. This can manifest as velopharyngeal insufficiency, which may result in dysphagia or dysarthria. The resultant hypernasal speech or nasopharyngeal regurgitation will peak within the first 2 weeks after injection and gradually subside thereafter.[7,9,15] However, because these effects are dose related, they may persist in patients with profound sensitivity to the toxin, or in patients who were administered higher than usual doses.

As previously discussed, one of the target muscles for BoNT injections is the TVP whose main function is opening of the eustachian tube and the subsequent equalization of middle ear pressure. By weakening the tensor, there may be resultant eustachian tube dysfunction. If these symptoms are severe, then they may be treated with pneumatic equalization tube placement. Diffusion or injection of the toxin into the palatopharyngeus muscle could result in weakening of the upward and anterior elevation of the pharynx contributing to dysphagia. Theoretical complications of bleeding or infection at the injection sites have not been reported in the literature.

11.5 Conclusion

Palatal myoclonus is an uncommon movement disorder affecting the pharynx. Medical management alone is rarely successful. The use of BoNT through localized injections into the TVP or LVP can relieve the symptoms with minimal risk and relatively low side effects. The effective use of BoNT is predicated upon comprehensive understanding of the toxin by the administering physician and extensive counseling with the patient regarding the typical cyclical nature of therapy with the toxin, its desired effects, and the potential undesired effects.

11.6 Key Points/Pearls

- Palatal myoclonus is synonymous with palatal tremor.
- Essential palatal tremor (EPT) presents with clicking tinnitus as a result of tensor veli palatini muscle contraction.
- Symptomatic palatal tremor (SPT) tends to involve the levator veli palatini muscle and can cause unwanted palatal movements.
- Extrapalatal neurological symptoms warrant full neurological workup.
- MRI imaging of the brain in SPT patients may show hypertrophic olivary degeneration.
- Botulinum neurotoxin (BoNT) injections directed at either muscle target are an effective local treatment.

- Adverse effects of BoNT in this region may include velopharyngeal insufficiency, dysphagia, and eustachian tube dysfunction.

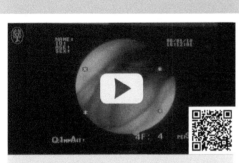

Video 11.1 Palatal myoclonus. With a transnasal endoscope in place, the irregular myoclonic jerks can be seen in the lateral aspect of soft palate and the palatopharyngeus muscle. The injection with EMG needle guidance is given transorally. A dose of 2.5 U/0.1 mL is given into the left side of the palate. [1:50]

References

[1] Zadikoff C, Lang AE, Klein C. The 'essentials' of essential palatal tremor: a reappraisal of the nosology. Brain.; 129(Pt 4): 832–840

[2] Sinclair CF, Gurey LE, Blitzer A. Palatal myoclonus: algorithm for management with botulinum toxin based on clinical disease characteristics. Laryngoscope.; 124(5):1164–1169

[3] Deuschl G, Toro C, Hallett M. Symptomatic and essential palatal tremor. 2. Differences of palatal movements. Mov Disord.; 9(6):676–678

[4] Deuschl G, Mischke G, Schenck E, Schulte-Mönting J, Lücking CH. Symptomatic and essential rhythmic palatal myoclonus. Brain.; 113(Pt 6):1645–1672

[5] Tilikete C, Desestret V. Hypertrophic olivary degeneration and palatal or oculopalatal tremor. Front Neurol.; 8:302

[6] Stamelou M, Saifee TA, Edwards MJ, Bhatia KP. Psychogenic palatal tremor may be underrecognized: reappraisal of a large series of cases. Mov Disord.; 27(9):1164–1168

[7] Varney SM, Demetroulakos JL, Fletcher MH, McQueen WJ, Hamilton MK. Palatal myoclonus: treatment with Clostridium botulinum toxin injection. Otolaryngol Head Neck Surg.; 114(2):317–320

[8] Bryce GE, Morrison MD. Botulinum toxin treatment of essential palatal myoclonus tinnitus. J Otolaryngol.; 27(4):213–216

[9] Jero J, Salmi T. Palatal myoclonus and clicking tinnitus in a 12-year-old girl–case report. Acta Otolaryngol Suppl.; 543: 61–62

[10] Srirompotong S, Tiamkao S, Jitpimolmard S. Botulinum toxin injection for objective tinnitus from palatal myoclonus: a case report. Journal of the Medical Association of Thailand.; 85(3):392–395

[11] Jamieson DR, Mann C, O'Reilly B, Thomas AM. Ear clicks in palatal tremor caused by activity of the levator veli palatini. Neurology.; 46(4):1168–1169

[12] Chien HF, Sanchez TG, Sennes LU, Barbosa ER. Endonasal approach of salpingopharyngeus muscle for the treatment of ear click related to palatal tremor. Parkinsonism Relat Disord.; 13(4):254–256

[13] Pirio Richardson S, Mari Z, Matsuhashi M, Hallett M. Psychogenic palatal tremor. Mov Disord.; 21(2):274–276

[14] Williams DR. Psychogenic palatal tremor. Mov Disord.; 19(3): 333–335

[15] Saeed SR, Brookes GB. The use of clostridium botulinum toxin in palatal myoclonus. A preliminary report. J Laryngol Otol.; 107(3):208–210

12

Botulinum Neurotoxin for Temporomandibular Disorders, Masseteric Hypertrophy, and Cosmetic Masseter Reduction

Michael Z. Lerner and Andrew Blitzer

Summary

Temporomandibular disorder (TMD) and associated masticatory muscle hyperfunction often result in a pain syndrome typically treated conservatively with diet modification, massage, and anti-inflammatory medications. For refractory cases, botulinum toxin injection into key muscle groups can offer relief from TMD pain. While botulinum toxin's analgesic properties remain incompletely understood, its action at the neuromuscular junction directly relieving muscle spasm and its potential inhibition of peripheral inflammatory peptide release are felt to be implicated. Workup focuses on patient selection, making sure to exclude those with arthrogenic forms of TMD and those in which botulinum toxin use might otherwise be contraindicated. Cosmetic masseteric reduction or iatrogenic atrophy can be achieved through targeted botulinum injection utilizing a similar injection technique.

Keywords: temporomandibular disorder, temporomandibular dysfunction, TMJ, muscles of mastication, masseter muscle, masseteric hypertrophy, cosmetic masseter reduction, pterygoid muscle

12.1 Introduction

Temporomandibular disorders (TMDs) describe a spectrum of disease affecting the temporomandibular joint and surrounding structures. It is estimated that between 5 and 12% of the U.S. population suffers from TMD-related symptoms.[1] Symptoms commonly include referred ear pain, headache, transmitted neck pain, decreased jaw mobility, pain while chewing, and crepitus with movement.[2] TMD-associated pain may arise from the joint itself (arthrogenic) or may be secondary to hyperfunction of the muscles of mastication (myofascial) resulting in chronic inflammation and pain.[3]

The myofascial form comprises the majority of TMD cases and may present by itself or in association with articular derangement. Etiologic factors include muscular spasticity secondary to malocclusion, bruxism, hypermobility, external stressors, and psychomotor behaviors such as excessive gum chewing.[4]

First-line pharmacologic treatment of TMD consists of anti-inflammatory agents, muscle relaxants, and tranquilizers. Physical treatments such as orthotic devices, physiotherapy, massage, acupuncture, and others are also often used. Other nonpharmacologic approaches include exercise, dietary adjustment, and biofeedback. Surgical interventions such as arthrocentesis, intra-articular steroid injection, arthroscopy, and open arthrotomy are rarely performed. Despite the myriad of treatment approaches, there is a lack of evidence that any one treatment is superior to another and additionally, a significant proportion of patients continue to have functional limitations and pain.[5]

Botulinum neurotoxin (BoNT) injection into the muscles of mastication represents a treatment option for those with TMD symptoms refractory to standard therapies. While the analgesic properties of BoNT are not completely understood, in the case of TMD, it is felt to be due to a combination of its action at the neuromuscular junction relieving masticatory muscle spasm and possibly a reduction in the release of inflammatory mediators such as calcitonin gene-related peptide, substance P, and glutamate, thus altering nociception.[6,7]

There have been several studies that collectively support the efficacy of BoNT for TMD. Schwartz and Freund[8] treated 46 patients with BoNT-A for TMD symptoms and assessed them at 2- and 8-week intervals for subjective pain, mean maximum voluntary contraction, interincisal oral opening, and tenderness to palpation. All patients demonstrated an improvement in all outcome measures except maximum voluntary contraction. Maximum voluntary contraction was reported to decrease after 2 weeks but then revert to baseline levels at 8 weeks. In an open-label study by Bentsianov et al,[4] the authors discovered a 70% response rate (defined as 50% reduction of severity and/or frequency of pain) when using BoNT injection into the masseter and temporalis muscles for TMD symptoms. Most recently, a randomized controlled pilot study of 20 patients by Patel et al[2]

showed that after incobotulinumtoxinA injection, there was a statistically significant reduction in pain and composite masticatory muscle tenderness score when compared to placebo saline injection.

12.2 Masseteric Hypertrophy and Cosmetic Masseter Reduction

Masseteric hypertrophy may occur due to an anatomic asymmetry of the jaw, habitual asymmetric use, clenching during exercise or sleep, or excessive chewing of gum.[4] Hypertrophy can be unilateral, resulting in an asymmetry of lateral face or bilateral, producing a square-jaw appearance.

Asian patients more frequently seek aesthetic alteration of hypertrophic masseter muscles to reduce a prominent mandibular angle. In fact, surgical reduction of the mandible is more common in Asia, despite the fact that botulinum toxin offers a less invasive treatment option. BoNT is ideal for patients with muscular hypertrophy rather than mandibular bony prominence as the source of lower face widening.[9]

12.3 Workup

12.3.1 Patient Selection

Patients should be at least 18 years of age and have had TMD symptoms for at least 3 months that have been refractory to conventional treatments for at least 6 weeks. The following patients should *not* be considered for BoNT therapy: patients with proven arthrogenic TMD, those who have had prior surgery for TMD, and patients using medications that have an effect at the neuromuscular junction or who have another disorder that interferes with neuromuscular function (e.g., myasthenia gravis).

Bentsianov et al[4] suggested using a visual analog scale (VAS) score greater than or equal to 4 but less than or equal to 9 on an 11-point scale as an additional patient selection criterion.

12.3.2 History and Physical Examination

A comprehensive history and physical examination with a focus on the head and neck is mandatory. It is important to include a dental history and examination as well. It is particularly important to ascertain if there is a history of psychological or psychiatric disorder, emotional stress, facial trauma, or poor dental care.

Symptoms associated with TMD include preauricular pain or otalgia, headaches, clicking, popping, or snapping of the jaw; limited range of mandibular movement and locking episodes; changes in occlusion; masticatory difficulty; and neck, shoulder, or back pain.

On physical examination, one should inspect for malocclusion, abnormal dental wear, missing teeth, and visible clenching or spasm of ipsilateral neck muscles. The temporomandibular joint should be palpated just below the zygomatic arch and 1 to 2 cm anterior to the tragus. Palpation should occur in both the open and closed positions. Determine the presence or absence of spasm, tenderness, and joint sound. Palpate the masseter, temporalis, pterygoids, and sternocleidomastoid muscles carefully.[7]

12.3.3 Laboratory Studies and Imaging

Blood work is usually unnecessary unless systemic illness is suspected, in which case a complete blood count, erythrocyte sedimentation rate, rheumatoid factor, and antinuclear antibody can be considered.

If the diagnosis is unclear from the history and physical examination alone, or medical management has been unsuccessful, imaging may also be considered. Conventional radiography is usually sufficient and may show erosion, sclerosis, or remodeling. Magnetic resonance imaging (MRI) and computed tomography (CT) are considered complementary modalities. MRI is superior for assessing the articular disk and soft-tissue structures of the temporomandibular joint, whereas CT is most useful for evaluating osseous changes, such as erosions, fracture, or postsurgical deformity.[10,11]

12.4 Anatomy

The temporomandibular joint is a synovial joint with articular surfaces on the condyle inferiorly, and articular tubercle and mandibular fossae of the squamous portion of the temporal bone superiorly. The articular surfaces are separated by an articular disk (or meniscus), which is a fibrocartilaginous structure providing a gliding surface for the condyle (▶ Fig. 12.1).

The adduction of the mandible (elevation or closing) is performed by the actions of the masseter (▶ Fig. 12.2), temporalis (▶ Fig. 12.3), and medial pterygoid (▶ Fig. 12.4). The mandible is actively abducted (depressed or opened) by the lateral pterygoids (▶ Fig. 12.5) and the supra- and infrahyoid musculature. Lateral excursion is allowed by actions of the contralateral pterygoids and masseter and the ipsilateral anterior portion of the temporalis muscles (▶ Table 12.1, ▶ Table 12.2).

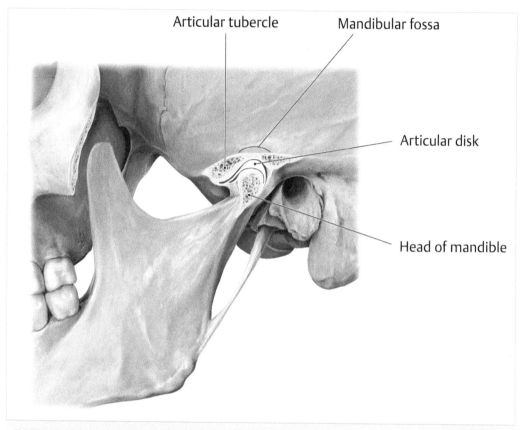

Fig. 12.1 Temporomandibular joint. (From Schuenke M, Schulte E, Schumacher U. THIEME Atlas of Anatomy: Head, Neck, and Neuroanatomy. Illustrations by Voll M and Wesker K. 2nd Ed. New York: Thieme Medical Publishers; 2016.)

12.5 Technique for Temporomandibular Disorders

A 27-gauge, hollow-bore, monopolar EMG electrode is placed into the muscle, which has been carefully palpated and identified prior to any procedure. The patient is first asked to activate the muscle ("bite down" in the case of the masseter) to verify correct placement of the needle. The intramuscular injection of the toxin is then initiated. The depth of injection approximates the belly of the muscle and should not be any deeper.

The required total dosage varies among patients, but we typically begin with a starting dose of 25 units (U) (100 U BoNT-A diluted with 2.0 mL of 0.9% sterile saline, resulting in a concentration of 5.0 U per 0.1 mL) to each masseter and temporalis muscle as symptoms dictate. This dose should be administered in five separate injections of 0.1 mL each of the aforementioned dilution, resulting in a total of 25 U in each individual muscle. The next scheduled dosage may be titrated up or down depending on the patient's response to the initial treatment. The origin of the temporalis muscle is the floor of the temporal fossa, and it inserts into the medial surface of the coronoid process and anterior border of the ramus. The patient is asked to identify the points of maximal tenderness within this area, and the 25 U BoNT-A is dispersed into the muscle at five of these points. Special care

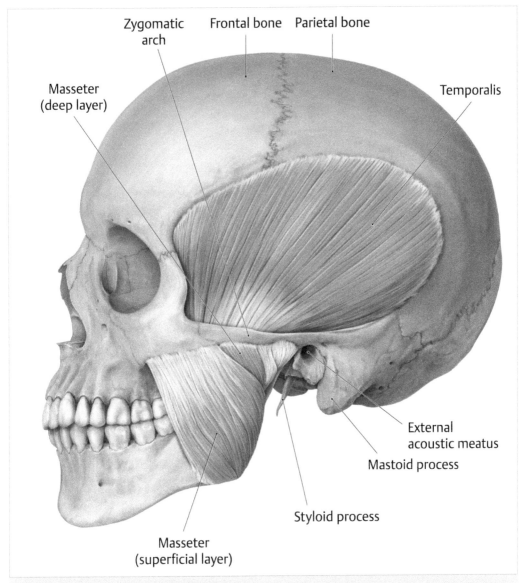

Zygomatic arch   Frontal bone   Parietal bone

Masseter (deep layer)

Temporalis

External acoustic meatus

Mastoid process

Styloid process

Masseter (superficial layer)

Fig. 12.2 Masseter muscle. (From Schuenke M, Schulte E, Schumacher U. THIEME Atlas of Anatomy: Head, Neck, and Neuroanatomy. Illustrations by Voll M and Wesker K. 2nd Ed. New York: Thieme Medical Publishers; 2016.)

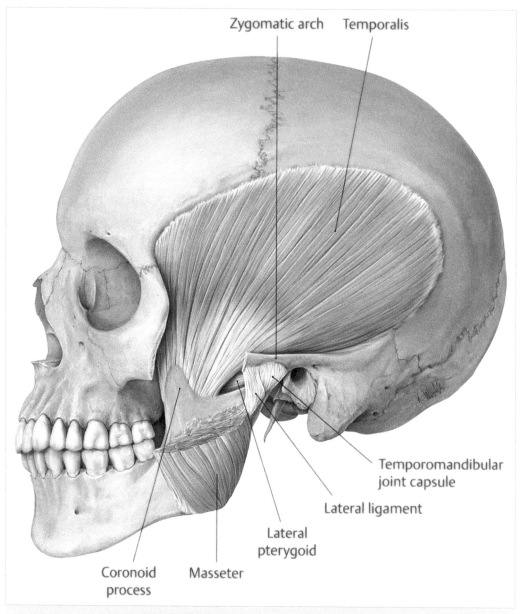

Fig. 12.3 Temporalis muscle. (From Schuenke M, Schulte E, Schumacher U. THIEME Atlas of Anatomy: Head, Neck, and Neuroanatomy. Illustrations by Voll M and Wesker K. 2nd Ed. New York: Thieme Medical Publishers; 2016.)

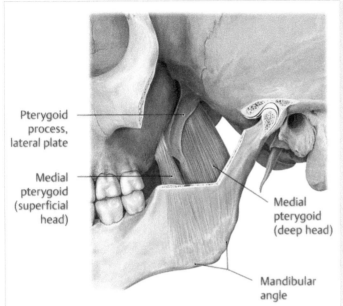

Fig. 12.4 Medial pterygoid. (From Schuenke M, Schulte E, Schumacher U. THIEME Atlas of Anatomy: Head, Neck, and Neuroanatomy. Illustrations by Voll M and Wesker K. 2nd Ed. New York: Thieme Medical Publishers; 2016.)

Pterygoid process, lateral plate

Medial pterygoid (superficial head)

Medial pterygoid (deep head)

Mandibular angle

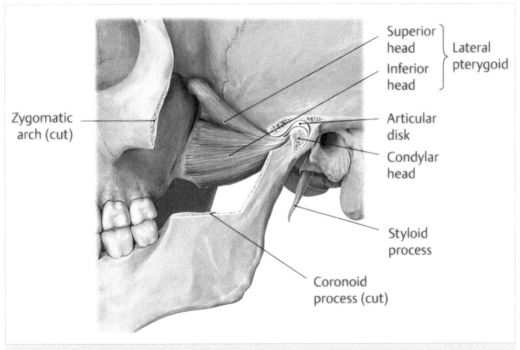

Superior head

Inferior head

Lateral pterygoid

Zygomatic arch (cut)

Articular disk

Condylar head

Styloid process

Coronoid process (cut)

Fig. 12.5 Lateral pterygoid. (From Schuenke M, Schulte E, Schumacher U. THIEME Atlas of Anatomy: Head, Neck, and Neuroanatomy. Illustrations by Voll M and Wesker K. 2nd Ed. New York: Thieme Medical Publishers; 2016.)

Table 12.1 Muscles of mastication: masseter and temporalis

Muscle	Origin	Insertion	Innervation	Action
Masseter	Superficial part: zygomatic arch (anterior two-thirds) Deep part: zygomatic arch (posterior one-third)	Mandibular angle (masseteric tuberosity)	Mandibular n. (cranial nerve V_3) via masseteric n.	Elevates (adducts) and protrudes mandible
Temporalis	Temporal fossa (inferior temporal line)	Coronoid process of mandible (apex and medial surface)	Mandibular n. (cranial nerve V_3) via deep temporal nn.	*Vertical fibers:* elevate (adduct) mandible *Horizontal fibers:* retract (retrude) mandible *Unilateral:* lateral movement of mandible (chewing)

Source: Adapted with permission from Gilroy AM, MacPherson BR, Ross LM. Atlas of Anatomy. New York, NY: Thieme; 2008:468.

Table 12.2 Muscles of mastication: pterygoid muscles

Muscle		Origin	Insertion	Innervation	Action
Lateral pterygoid	Superior head	Greater wing of sphenoid bone (infratemporal crest)	Temporomandibular joint (articular disk)	Mandibular n. (cranial nerve V_3) via lateral pterygoid n.	*Bilateral:* protrudes mandible (pulls articular disk forward)
	Inferior head	Lateral pterygoid plate (lateral surface)	Mandible (condylar process)		*Unilateral:* lateral movements of mandible (chewing)
Medial pterygoid	Superficial head	Maxilla (tuberosity)	Pterygoid tuberosity on medial surface of the mandibular angle	Mandibular n. (cranial nerve V_3) via medial pterygoid n.	Elevates (adducts) mandible
	Deep head	Medial surface of lateral pterygoid plate and pterygoid fossa			

Source: Adapted with permission from Gilroy AM, MacPherson BR, Ross LM. Atlas of Anatomy. New York, NY: Thieme; 2008:469.

should be taken to avoid the superficial temporal vessels, which can cause unnecessary and unsightly postinjection ecchymosis if injured (▶ Fig. 12.6).

The origin of the masseter muscle is the inferior border of the zygomatic arch. The insertion is onto the lateral surface of the ramus and coronoid process. The injections may be routed trans-cutaneously or intraorally, with the former being utilized more often. Again, a total of 25 U should be injected into each individual muscle, using five separate injections of 0.1 mL each (of 5 U/0.1 mL BoNT-A solution). Injection sites should be based on the patient's prior identification of the areas of maximal discomfort (▶ Fig. 12.7).

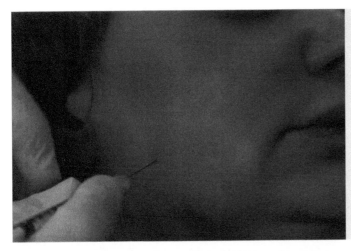

Fig. 12.6 Masseter muscle injection.

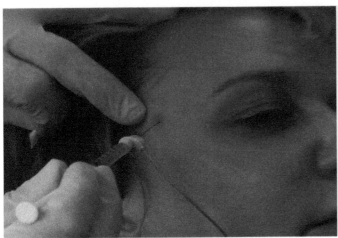

Fig. 12.7 Temporalis muscle injection.

Treatment of the lateral or external pterygoid is most beneficial for patients who have as their primary symptom teeth grinding or severe lateral excursion. This injection should be given intraorally under EMG guidance. The lateral pterygoid plate is palpated, and the needle is placed between this plate and the coronoid process of the mandible. The needle should be oriented parallel to the length of the muscle. Once the needle is in position, the patient is asked to produce lateral excursions of the jaw as a confirmatory gesture and bursts of motor endplate potentials will be noted. The starting dose for each pterygoid muscle is typically 7.5 U per muscle (2.5 U/0.1 mL

solution created by diluting 100 U BoNT-A with 4.0 mL of 0.9% sterile saline)[4] (▶ Fig. 12.8).

12.6 Technique for Masseteric Hypertrophy and Cosmetic Masseter Reduction

Muscles may be treated in a manner similar to that reported for TMD. Generally, for cosmetic reduction of the masseters, 25 U of BoNT-A is injected into the muscle in an area posterior to a line drawn from lateral orbital rim through facial notch and inferior to a line drawn from tragus of the ear to the corner of the mouth—this will deliver the toxin to the bulk of inferior muscle and prevent diffusion to the facial mimetic muscles. Patients are reevaluated at 2 weeks, and additional toxin may be added if deemed necessary (▶ Fig. 12.9).

Where there is asymmetry, 25 U is injected in five positions of the hypertrophied muscle and 10 U is injected contralaterally to prevent shifting hyperfunction to the opposite side. In cases where there

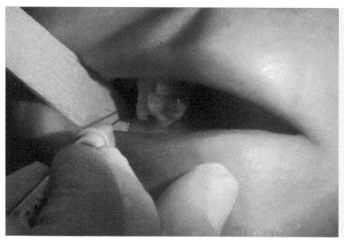

Fig. 12.8 Lateral pterygoid muscle injection.

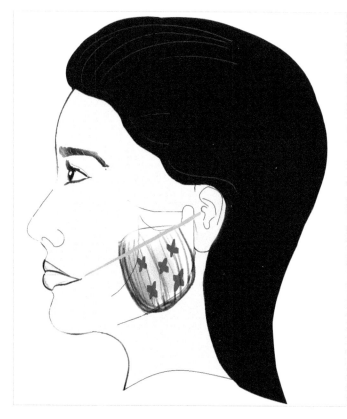

Fig. 12.9 Areas of injection of cosmetic masseter reduction.

is bilateral hypertrophy, an equal dose is delivered to each muscle.

12.7 Follow-up

Patients may be evaluated at 2 weeks to assess the success of treatment. Patients should report any adverse effects. If pain or enlargement persists, the clinician may elect to add additional toxin to the affected areas.

12.8 Complications and Pitfalls

The primary complications associated with injection of the masseter, temporalis, and lateral pterygoid are discussed in Chapter 5. The main adverse effect usually relates to excessive weakening of the masticatory muscles such that chewing becomes difficult. If this complication does occur, the patient should be reassured that chewing will return to baseline once the toxin wears off. Muscle wasting may also occur with repeated injections. Injection site pain is possible, but infrequently reported. Another uncommon complication is perioral facial weakness secondary to toxin diffusion to the zygomaticus major muscle. Generally, complications are infrequent and the procedure is well tolerated by most patients.

12.9 Key Points/Pearls

- For carefully selected patients with temporomandibular disorder, botulinum neurotoxin is a safe and effective treatment option that may augment the efficacy of both traditional conservative measures and surgical interventions.
- Further research is required to establish specific selection criteria.

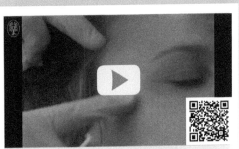

Video 12.1 Temporomandibular disorders. (**a**) Masseter muscle injection: given with a hollow-bore EMG needle. Five sites are injected with 2.5 to 5 U/0.1 mL of Botox in each muscle. Once the needle is inserted, the patient is instructed to clench teeth to elicit activity. (**b**) Temporalis muscle injection: the areas of tenderness are elicited by palpation. In this patient, three areas in the anterior portion of the muscle are injected with 2.5 U/0.1 mL of Botox. (**c**) External pterygoid muscle injection: this muscle is best reached with EMG control with an intraoral approach. This allows the toxin to be accurately place along the length of the muscle. The patient is asked to move her jaw side to side to activate the muscle. [1:51]

References

[1] Schiffman E, Ohrbach R, Truelove E, et al. International RDC/TMD Consortium Network, International association for Dental Research, Orofacial Pain Special Interest Group, International Association for the Study of Pain. Diagnostic criteria for temporomandibular disorders (DC/TMD) for clinical and research applications: recommendations of the International RDC/TMD Consortium Network and Orofacial Pain Special Interest Group. J Oral Facial Pain Headache.; 28(1):6–27

[2] Patel AA, Lerner MZ, Blitzer A. IncobotulinumtoxinA injection for temporomandibular joint disorder: a randomized controlled pilot study. Ann Otol Rhinol Laryngol.; 126(4):328–333

[3] Mohl ND, Ohrbach R. Clinical decision making for temporomandibular disorders. J Dent Educ.; 56(12):823–833

[4] Bentsianov B, Francis A, Blitzer A. Botulinum toxin treatment of temporomandibular disorders, masseteric hypertrophy, and cosmetic masseter reduction. Oper Tech Otolaryngol-Head Neck Surg.; 15(2):110–113

[5] Zenz M, Strumpf M, Tryba M. Long-term oral opioid therapy in patients with chronic nonmalignant pain. J Pain Symptom Manage.; 7(2):69–77

[6] Song PC, Schwartz J, Blitzer A. The emerging role of botulinum toxin in the treatment of temporomandibular disorders. Oral Dis.; 13(3):253–260

[7] Bossowska A, Lepiarczyk E, Mazur U, Janikiewicz P, Markiewicz W. Botulinum toxin type A induces changes in the chemical coding of substance P-immunoreactive dorsal root ganglia sensory neurons supplying the porcine urinary bladder. Toxins (Basel).; 7(11):4797–4816

[8] Schwartz M, Freund B. Treatment of temporomandibular disorders with botulinum toxin. Clin J Pain.; 18(6) Suppl:S198–S203

[9] Ahn J, Horn C, Blitzer A. Botulinum toxin for masseter reduction in Asian patients. Arch Facial Plast Surg.; 6(3):188–191

[10] Roth C, Ward RJ, Tsai S, Zolotor W, Tello R. MR imaging of the TMJ: a pictorial essay. Appl Radiol.; 34:9–16

[11] Boeddinghaus R, Whyte A. Computed tomography of the temporomandibular joint. J Med Imaging Radiat Oncol.; 57(4):448–454

13
Botulinum Neurotoxin Therapy in the Laryngopharynx

Craig H. Zalvan, Phillip C. Song, Nwanmegha Young, and Andrew Blitzer

Summary

The use of botulinum toxin in the larynx has been well established for disorders such as spasmodic dysphonia and cricopharyngeal dysfunction. In addition to these laryngeal presentations, botulinum toxin can be used for a myriad of other laryngopharyngeal presentations including but not limited to muscle tension dysphonia, laryngeal tremor, paradoxical vocal fold motion (frequently referred to as vocal cord dysfunction), spastic dysarthria, arytenoid rebalancing, idiopathic chronic cough, and contact granulomas. This chapter will review the literature and experience of the authors with the use of botulinum toxin in treating these disorders.

Keywords: vocal fold paralysis, cough, tic, arytenoid, TEP, nodules, puberphonia, granuloma, stenosis

13.1 Introduction

For over 30 years, botulinum neurotoxin (BoNT) has been the gold-standard treatment for spasmodic dysphonia. Since it was first publicized in mainstream society, the use of BoNT has grown at a staggering rate, with toxin being utilized in almost every field of medicine. Within the field of laryngology, the use of BoNT has also found a multitude of uses other than for spasmodic dysphonia. Almost any type of hyperkinetic or compensatory behavior found can be treated with the use of this toxin with a high degree of success, a low side-effect profile, and significant patient satisfaction. Toxin has been injected into the laryngopharynx for vocal tics, stuttering, vocal tremor, ventricular dysphonia, bilateral vocal fold paralysis, tracheoesophageal speech failure, as well as many other applications. By using toxin, many of these symptoms are controlled more easily, often requiring less systemic medication. Also, toxin is used as an adjunct to other types of traditional therapy, such as voice therapy and swallowing therapy, and even to surgical interventions. Additionally, because of the physiologic effects of weakening muscle, the toxin can be used to "rebalance" the larynx. In cases of bilateral vocal fold paresis, selectively weakening the adductor muscles can provide an adequate airway and help avoid a surgical intervention. Patients with vocal fold granulomas can benefit from toxin injection to help decrease the traumatic forces of the posterior glottis, thus decreasing the recurrence of granuloma and helping with resolution of persistent granulomas. In almost every situation of hyperfunction of the laryngeal and extralaryngeal musculature, BoNT can be used to help ameliorate symptoms and provide significant, reproducible relief for patients.

As with most patients presenting with hyperfunctional disorders of the larynx, the primary diagnostic modality is laryngoscopy with or without strobo-scopy. A detailed evaluation of the laryng-opharyngeal structures demonstrates any abnormalities of function, including laryngeal closure, pharyngeal contrac-tion, vocal fold motion, and laryngeal elevation. Additionally, anatomic abnor-malities are visualized, indicating such findings as benign vocal fold mucosal dis-ease, vocal fold granulomas, and excessive muscular tension. Typically, no further workup is necessary other than a thor-ough history and a physical examination of the head and neck.

Although BoNT may be very successful for a variety of hyperkinetic laryngeal disorders, care must be taken to evaluate the larynx in a systematic and critical manner. We have used selective chemo-denervation for a variety of conditions such as muscle tension dysphonia, laryngeal tremor, paradoxical vocal fold motion (frequently referred to as vocal cord dysfunction), spastic dysarthria, arytenoid rebalancing, idiopathic chronic cough, and contact granulomas, and results can be variable. The following considerations should accompany the decision-making process when consider-ing selective laryngeal chemodenervation using BoNT in these less common laryng-eal disorders.

1. The specificity of injections may be inadequate due to inherent difficulties with site localization and the inevita-ble diffusion of BoNT to adjacent muscles within the relatively narrow injection field of the larynx.

2. Diagnostic criteria and our ability to determine the root cause of some laryngeal disorders with existing technology is an inexact science. Clinical examination and visualization during phonation is a rough guide to laryngeal activity. Visualization of the larynx with the endoscope allows a single angle of view that limits evalua-tion of inferior and deeper structures. In the case of muscle tension dysphonia and vocal hyperfunction, the true vocal folds are often obscured by the function of the supraglottic structures. Other tools such as laryngeal electromyogra-phy (LEMG) may be a more sensitive instrument; however, in its current state, LEMG is still an imprecise tool. The technique to perform EMG-guided injection of BoNT has been described extensively in Chapter 6.

3. A variety of dysfunction produces the same clinical appearance. For instance, muscle tension dysphonia can be the end result of hyperfunction of certain laryngeal muscle groups, hypofunction of others, paresis, poor coordination, inadequate or disruptive sensory feedback, or anatomic pathology.

4. A well-defined management algorithm incorporating selective chemodenerva-tion for these conditions does not exist. Individual practitioners are using BoNT without a clear constructive clinical model, resulting in a wide range of injection techniques and therapies. Instead of treating botulinum injections like a surgical tool, it is perceived as a medication with a specific pharmaco-logic action. BoNT should be viewed as an instrument with properties of cutting or severing a nerve. In this chapter, we discuss our general experi-ence and collective expertise with these disorders; however, use of this "chemi-cal knife" correctly requires an individ-ualized plan of care and treatment.

5. Response to treatment is gauged by the outcome of the voice, resolution of the dysfunction, granuloma, or cough. Our guidelines are meant as suggestive dosing which may vary depending on severity of the symptom. If the initial injection fails to improve the symptom and there are no significant side effects, a repeat injection can be performed typically with one half the dose.

13.2 Bilateral Vocal Fold Paralysis

Bilateral vocal fold paralysis can be a devastating consequence of neck surgery, brainstem disease, or systemic disease that often leaves a patient with severe debilitation including shortness of breath and stridor with airway compromise. It is imperative to differentiate bilateral cricoarytenoid joint ankylosis or posterior glottic web as a complication of intubation from true bilateral vocal fold paralysis. Laryngeal EMG followed by examination under anesthesia to evaluate for posterior glottic stenosis (PGS) and/or cricoarytenoid joint ankylosis, if EMG is normal, is an effective technique to establish the correct diagnosis. Patients often require airway intervention ranging from suture lateralization, simple posterior vocal fold cordotomy, or tracheotomy. While some laryngologists advocate waiting for at least 1 year from the onset of the bilateral immobility before performing a destructive laryngeal procedure to create an adequate airway to allow for laryngeal patency and removal of a tracheotomy tube, others intervene sooner if signs of chronic denervation are present on laryngeal EMG, or if the mechanism of injury suggests poor prognosis. However, when patients have bilateral vocal paresis with possible return of function given the mechanism or favorable EMG findings, alternative treatments with BoNT are considered. Nimodipine is a promising adjunctive treatment that has been shown to increase the likelihood of neural regeneration, although multicenter human studies have not yet been performed.[1]

Many patients who are newly diagnosed with airway compromise due to bilateral paresis or paralysis may be stable at rest or moderately symptomatic without distress. In this situation, a tracheotomy can possibly be avoided, removed early, or capped, by using BoNT injection into either unilateral or bilateral thyroarytenoid and lateral cricoarytenoid (TA/LCA) muscle complex. By inhibiting the adductory function during reinnervation, the abductor muscles can contract unopposed, often leading to a larger airway caliber that allows for better airflow. In one study, 10 of 11 patients obtained substantial relief from airway obstruction after either bilateral or unilateral followed by bilateral BoNT injection into the TA/LCA complex which can result in increased airway patency at rest and with activity.[2]

In addition to injecting the TA/LCA complex, recent intervention has focused on the cricothyroid muscles. In a pediatric case series, a small incision to expose the cricothyroid muscles with subsequent direct intramuscular injection of 4 to 10 units (U) of BoNT resulted with decannulation of five of six patients, with a larger airway caliber reported postinjection.[3] A small adult series of three patients using transcutaneous cricothyroid muscle injections of BoNT ranging from 2.5 to 3 U was used to treat their bilateral vocal fold paralysis with success in avoiding tracheotomy and alleviating symptoms of dyspnea.[4]

Another use of BoNT in patients with bilateral vocal fold paralysis pertains to those with implantable laryngeal stimulators within the posterior cricoarytenoid (PCA) muscle. By weakening the opposing adductory forces with chemical denervation, the airway patency was increased, alleviating the symptoms of dyspnea. Thus, by using electrical stimulation and chemical denervation, this group was able to decannulate patients with longstanding bilateral vocal fold paralysis.[5]

Typical treatment utilizing BoNT involves bilateral injections of the thyroarytenoid muscles utilizing the standard EMG-guided anterior neck approach; 2.5 U of toxin is injected bilaterally as the initial dose. A second dose of 0.5 to 1 U can be injected 2 to 3 weeks after the initial dose if there has been little or no response. Typical side effects can range from no ill effects to severe breathiness and occasional coughing while drinking liquids. Gross aspiration is possible but has not occurred in our experience. Patients with severe airway compromise or progressive compromise despite BoNT injection are not good candidates for this type of medical intervention, and airway security is the primary concern.

13.3 Tracheoesophageal Speech Failure

Loss of voice after total laryngectomy is an unavoidable morbidity. However, with the widespread use of a tracheoesophageal puncture (TEP) and voice prosthesis, patients can develop and maintain the ability to communicate. A major disappointment occurs when that ability is lost again because of dysfunction of the prosthesis from fungal infection, dislodgement, and hyperfunction of the cricopharyngeus (even if CP myotomy was performed at the time of the laryngectomy), or pharyngoesophageal segment, preventing normal airflow through the TEP. In addition, some laryngectomy patients initially fail an insufflation test of the pharyngoesophageal segment, demonstrating hyperfunction of this segment and likely poor TEP function.

The use of BoNT had been shown to be an excellent adjunct in the treatment of these hyperfunctional disorders of the pharyngoesophageal segment. By paralyzing the hyperfunctional muscle fibers, airflow through the TEP and pharyngoesophageal segment is enhanced, resulting in fluent esophageal speech. In cases where the etiology of failure of the TEP is uncertain, BoNT injection into the inferior constrictor and cricopharyngeal fibers can provide diagnostic information by either its success or failure. If successful at ameliorating the problem, BoNT can also be administered for long-term treatment. BoNT may be administered transcutaneously to the suprastomal region using EMG guidance, although scar tissue often prevents robust signal; 50 U is the typical starting dose delivered bilaterally in equal doses. The injection can also be performed without EMG, if the plunger of the syringe is withdrawn prior to injection to prevent inadvertent intravascular or intraluminal injection. The practitioner should be aware of the medialized position of the carotid arteries following total laryngectomy. If there is no response, up to another 50 U can then be administered. The cricopharyngeus muscle is identified by finding baseline activity at rest, which diminishes with a swallow with prompt return of function after the swallow.[6] Side effects are rare and may include some dysphagia from weakened constrictor muscles from toxin diffusion. Because of the alaryngeal state, there is no risk of aspiration or airway compromise.

13.4 Benign Vocal Fold Disease

Benign vocal fold disease such as vocal fold nodules, polyps, cysts, granulomas, and hemorrhages all share a common etiologic factor: trauma. Chronic overuse of the voice, vocal abuse, acute phonatory trauma from coughing and yelling, and excessive Valsalva maneuver can all lead to thickening of the epithelium of the vocal folds, subepithelial fibrosis, and vocal hemorrhage. In many of these cases, voice therapy is the gold standard of treatment. Other cases require microsurgical intervention using a microflap technique of removal to optimize vocal outcome. However, often patients are reluctant to undergo surgery, and surgery does entail some small risk of long-term dysphonia. In certain circumstances, in patients with recurrent vocal fold benign disease, or dysphonia that persists despite voice therapy and surgery, BoNT can be used as an adjunct to temporarily weaken the adductor forces of the glottis to allow for healing or resolution of the benign vocal fold disease. By using this technique, there is no risk to the superficial lamina propria from surgical trauma. In addition, patients can continue undergoing voice therapy to help prevent recurrent lesions. Some patients can develop a temporary breathiness inherent in injecting the adductor muscles with BoNT. Though typically temporary, these periods of breathiness can be decreased by serial injections of lower doses of BoNT. The typical starting dose is 0.5 U of toxin delivered by EMG-guided injection into the thyroarytenoid muscle. If no change in voice is noted, an additional booster of 0.5 U can be attempted. Side effects are typical for BoNT injection and include breathiness and possible aspiration. Mild breathiness for a few weeks is ideal, as this gives time for the mucosal pathology to resolve. With ongoing voice therapy, these lesions can actually regress and often do not recur once behavioral changes have been made.

13.5 Muscle Tension Dysphonia

The success of BoNT for treating primary muscle tension dysphonia (noncompensatory) is based on proper and critical evaluation of larynx function to identify laryngeal pathology as well as analysis of laryngeal behavior to distinguish between compensatory and primary hyperfunction. Coordination with a trusted and experienced voice therapist is very important. BoNT injections are considered for those patients with severe symptoms who have failed voice therapy. Ongoing voice therapy is necessary because the BoNT injections are temporary, and long-lasting improvement depends on functional changes in laryngeal behavior. The injections can be considered a temporary chemical "splint" that forces reduction in hyperfunctional behavior. However, until the patient understands and can control the behavior, the voice symptoms are likely to return. In fact, there may be a danger in exacerbating the symptoms if the behavior is exaggerated or new dysfunctional compensatory strategies develop. An additional usage of BoNT would be to unload the larynx to reveal laryngeal pathology that was previously not seen secondary to the hyperfunction, that is, glottic pathology that could not be evaluated due to false vocal fold compression during phonation.

Pacheco et al described a series of seven patients who underwent injection of BoNT into their ventricular folds in the operating room. Of the six patients who were followed up, five showed improvement based on pretreatment and posttreatment GRBAS (grade, roughness, breathiness, asthenia, strain) scores.[7] In our experience, the area and dose of injection can vary based on the clinical evaluation of the larynx and determination of the hyperfunctional muscles.

Given the false vocal folds are relatively devoid of muscle, the effect is likely from diffusion of the BoNT to the intrinsic musculature. Another approach would be to inject a smaller dose of BoNT into the LCA and possibly into the extrinsic, strap muscles. 0.5 U into the LCA and 2 to 3 U in the overlying strap muscle is the typical starting dose. Traditional voice therapy following the injection of BoNT is useful in the rehabilitation process.

13.6 Evaluation

It is critical to ascertain which laryngeal muscles are dysfunctional. There are several ways to categorize types of laryngeal muscle tension dysphonia. Supraglottic manifestations of hyperfunction include ventricular hyperfunction, which is over-closure of the false vocal folds over the true ones; anterior posterior compression, which refers to overclosure secondary to the epiglottis and arytenoid complex narrowing; and sphincteric closure, in which both dimensions are incorporated, closing off the larynx. Muscle tension may also be the product of excessive tension of the vocal folds without significant supra-glottic activity. There may be overrotation of the LCA, creating a posterior glottic gap and excessive protrusion of the vocalis process. There may also be excessive crico-thyroid muscle motion leading to a lengthened and tight vocal fold. Additionally, hyperfunction of the transverse aryte-noid muscle could result with a scissoring action of the posterior glottis.

13.7 Botulinum Therapy

For lateral hyperfunction or hyperfunc-tion causing predominantly lateral hyper-function, excessive length and tension of the true vocal folds, the TA and LCA are the most commonly addressed groups of muscles. LCA hyperfunction can be manifested by overrotation of the posteri-or glottis, forming a prominence of the vocalis process or a Y-shaped posterior glottal gap. If it is determined to be signif-icant hyperfunction of the cricothyroid muscle, as manifested by increased pitch, a lengthened vocal fold, and tension/pain in the cricothyroid visor, cricothyroid injections should be tried. Interarytenoid injections can also be given in cases where overactive transverse arytenoids muscles are suspected.

BoNT injections can be performed on the larynx via transcutaneous EMG-guided methods. A good starting dose for treating muscle tension dysphonia is about 2.5 to 5.0 U per side in the office setting and up to 30 U per side in the operating room without EMG guidance. The dose is higher than our standard initial dose for spasmodic dysphonia. The patient should have some breathiness and loss of projection after the injection. Possible side effects include dysphagia (typically coughing and choking on thin liquids), odynophagia, local injection site reactions such as bruising and bleeding, and a very slight chance of regional diffusion of the Botox into other sites.

13.8 Puberphonia

Puberphonia or mutational falsetto is a hyperfunctional vocal disorder that afflicts primarily teenage boys. The underlying condition is the retention of the prepubes-cent voice after puberty. This may be secondary to a "nonacceptance" of the new, mature, male voice or a regression back to prepubescent vocal patterns, resulting in a high-pitched, feminized, or androgynous voice pattern. As with all laryngeal applications for BoNT, care must be taken to identify and correct the hyper-functional muscle groups and rule out structural vocal fold problems, notably sulcus and glottal insufficiency.

The first line of treatment is always with an experienced voice pathologist who has expertise in the treatment of puberphonia. BoNT treatment may be indicated for patients with puberphonia who have failed voice therapy. Psychiatric evaluation to identify and treat emotional or cognitive obstacles to the acceptance of the mature voice may be necessary prior to the procedure, especially in cases of regression and in older patients. For teenagers, the main problem may be physiologic adjustment difficulties during the transitional stages of laryngeal development.

The evaluation of puberphonia is similar to that of muscle tension dysphonia: identify the laryngeal muscle groups that are dysfunctional. Typically, the voice is high-pitched and strained. The cricothyroid and strap muscles are hyperfunctional with elevated tension along the vocal folds and a larynx that is in a "high" position. Palpation of the cricothyroid visor and the thyrohyoid space can elucidate these muscles. The laryngoscopy and stroboscopy should reflect the hyperfunctional behavior and be clear of other laryngeal disease. Ongoing voice therapy is important to help maintain the homeostasis.

In our experience, transcutaneous EMG-guided BoNT directed at the cricothyroid muscle and at the TA/LCA complex is generally the most successful treatment. The cricothyroid muscles can be identified with the EMG needle inserted lateral to the cricothyroid space, with the needle directed superficial to the cricoid lamina toward the lateral thyroid lamina. The starting dose is 5.0 mouse units per side. The patient is directed to begin phonation at the lowest pitch and perform a pitch glide into falsetto. With puberphonia, the EMG discharge is typically at the onset of phonation because the cricothyroid muscle is discharged even at the lower pitch range. The TA/LCA complex is treated with 2.5 to 5.0 mouse units, as is typical for other muscle tension disorders.

13.9 Tourette Syndrome and Laryngeal Tics

Tourette syndrome and laryngeal tics are neuropsychiatric disorders of uncontrollable motor and phonic impulses. For simple motor tics, there does seem to be an improvement in the frequency and premonitory or urge symptoms associated with the motor spasms. Manifestations of Tourette syndrome tend to be complex motor behaviors, and laryngeal Botox may be beneficial in reducing the loudness and volume of the vocalizations as well as in decreasing the frequency. The phonic tics may be short, brief involuntary movements or vocalizations. They are repetitive, but not regular or rhythmic in nature. The vocalizations can be simple (sniff, bark, throat clearing, or cough) or complex (echolalia, palilalia, and coprolalia). There is a significant association with psychiatric disorders such as attention deficit hyperactivity disorder, obsessive compulsive disorder, and autism.

There has been one randomized prospective trial on the efficacy of BoNT for simple motor tics in the head and neck.[8] In this study of 18 patients using BoNT in a variety of sites in the head and neck, the authors demonstrated an average reduction of 37% in tic frequency based on videotaped assessment as compared with saline injection.

BoNT is considered an adjuvant symptomatic treatment. Primary pharmacologic treatment for Tourette syndrome is based on functional disability. Treatment can range from simple observation and treatment of comorbid psychiatric conditions to neuroleptic agents, primarily dopamine receptor blockers. Clonidine, guanfacine, clonazepam, and baclofen have been used for tic suppression with variable success; however, side effects often limit their utility. BoNT to the larynx can be useful for reduction and suppression in the volume and frequency of the involuntary vocalizations presumably by weakening the muscles driving the tic behavior and potentially the premonitory urge that drives them.[9]

To reduce loudness and volume, BoNT is injected into the TA/LCA complex via transcutaneous EMG-guided method. The starting dose is usually 2.5 U per side and is higher than that used for spasmodic dysphonia. A weak, breathy, and asthenic voice is considered a natural part of the therapy.

13.10 Vocal Process Granulomas

Laryngeal granulomas are abnormal rests of wound healing tissue composed of fibroblasts that most often arise in the posterior aspects of the vocal folds along the vocal process. Also described as contact granulomas and contact erosions, these lesions are traumatic and inflammatory in nature, with a high degree of association with vocal hyperfunction and laryngopharyngeal reflux. The clinical behavior of these lesions ranges from indolent to aggressive, and symptoms are usually related to size. Small granulomas may be asymptomatic, whereas larger granulomas can result in dysphonia, dysphagia, and airway obstruction.

Although contact granulomas that arise after intubation or trauma (postintubation granulomas) often disappear with observation or treatment with antireflux therapy, idiopathic granulomas have high rates of recurrence after removal, and surgery alone is not considered an effective means of treatment.[10] These lesions are primarily managed medically, with voice rest, inhaled or intralesional steroid treatments, voice therapy, and antireflux

therapy. BoNT alone or in conjunction with other treatments can be used as a chemical splint to reduce phonotrauma along the vocal process keeping the posterior vocal folds more lateralized.[11,12]

The utility of BoNT injections in the larynx for vocalis process granulomas depends on the clinical evaluation of the etiology of the disease and the degree of laryngeal hyperfunction. Damrose and Damrose[13] reported their experiences using laryngeal BoNT injection for refractory laryngeal granulomas in seven patients. They reported success in all seven of the treated patients using doses ranging from 10 to 25 U divided into both vocal folds. In our experience, BoNT injections have a high rate of initial success; however, long-term success often requires continued acid suppression therapy and changes in vocal behavior.

BoNT injections in the presence of compensatory hyperfunction for glottal incompetence, such as that associated with sulcus vocalis, loss of superficial lamina propria, vocal fold paresis, or presbylarynges, are more likely to fail, even with adequate voice therapy. In these cases, the posterior glottis undergoes excessive trauma in order for the patient to maintain a functional voice. Vocal fold augmentation to address the underlying glottal insufficiency may be used in these cases to reduce posterior glottal striking forces.[14]

BoNT delivered for the treatment of laryngeal granulomas undergoes similar evaluation as for primary muscle tension dysphonia. The most common injection sites are the TA/LCA complex and the interarytenoid muscles. The TA/LCA complex is treated with 2.5 to 5.0 mouse units, as is typical for other muscle tension disorders. In our hands, the interarytenoid injection is generally administered under direct visualization and a transcutaneous approach either superiorly through the thyrohyoid membrane or inferiorly through the cricothyroid membrane. The needle is seen traversing the glottic airspace and between 10 and 20 mouse units are injected into the interarytenoid region. Care must be taken not to insert the needle too deep, or it may infiltrate into the PCA.

The TA/LCA injections may also be performed visually through the same approach.

13.11 Posterior Glottic Stenosis

A severe consequence of trauma to the vocal process and interarytenoid mucosa is the development of PGS and interarytenoid synechia. Vocal process granulomas (VPG) and contact erosions that arise after intubation or trauma (postintubation granulomas) usually resolve with observation or treatment with antireflux therapy. However, abnormal wound healing response in the posterior glottis can result in PGS with bilateral vocal fold immobility, glottic fixation, airway distress, and tracheostomy dependence. The development of PGS has been associated with prolonged intubation, large ETT, and medical factors such as diabetes and ischemia.[15] Substantial posterior bilateral erosions, mucosal ulcerations of the interarytenoid region, and diminished abduction of the vocal folds should raise suspicion for the development of PGS.

BoNT injections may have a role in reducing the progressive adduction and medial fibrosis of the vocal folds in PGS. Injection of the interarytenoid region and the TA/LCA muscles have the potential to distract the vocal folds laterally. The technique is described in the granuloma section. Thyroarytenoid and interarytenoid BoNT injections can also be performed in the operating room in conjunction with surgical lateralization techniques such as partial arytenoidectomy and PGS lysis with posterior mucosal grafting.[16]

13.12 Arytenoid Rebalancing

Arytenoid rebalancing with BoNT for the treatment of arytenoid dislocation has been described sporadically in the literature.[17] Arytenoid dislocation is often difficult to diagnose as the position of the arytenoid can be quite variable. Typically, anterior arytenoid dislocation produces a lax, bowed vocal fold with a medialized and anterior displacement of the arytenoid body, and there is often an absent "jostle" sign. The anterior dislocation lowers the vocalis process, producing a vertical mismatch that adds to the degree of glottal incompetence. This position is also common in the paralyzed vocal fold. There may be a line of demarcation at the junction of the cricoid and arytenoids in cases of complete dislocation. The posterior arytenoid dislocation results in a posterior and laterally positioned arytenoid with a taut vocal fold. In either case, the arytenoid is immobile and glottic incompetence is common. Evidence of supraglottic contraction may help in differentiating between dislocation and paralysis. The diagnosis usually requires manual palpation or the arytenoids, radiographic evidence of the arytenoid dislocation, and/ or laryngeal EMG. Operative treatment to relocate the arytenoid by closed reduction is the most common practice. This is often attempted during direct laryngoscopy by pushing the arytenoids back over the cricoid ledge. However, surgical success producing arytenoid mobility and reestablishing glottic competence is rare. BoNT has been advocated as an adjuvant treatment to rebalance the arytenoid to guide it to a more functional position.

BoNT injections have also been used as a surgical adjunct after repair of an avulsed vocal process. Vocal process avulsion is associated with laryngeal trauma which results in a separation of the vocal process from the body of the arytenoid cartilage and can be associated with anterior arytenoid dislocation and subluxation. After surgical repair, BoNT can be administered to the TA/LCA muscles to reduce muscle motion which may disrupt the suture line.[18]

In an anteriorly displaced arytenoid, the PCA muscle is often torn or excessively lax because of the traumatic stretch injury. The treatment rationale is to rebalance the arytenoids on top of the cricoid ledge by weakening the adductor groups. The common targets are the interarytenoid muscles and the TA/LCA complex. This would produce a relative strengthening of the abductor (the PCA), resulting in a more posterior arytenoid position. This can be performed during the surgical relocation attempt in the operating room or afterward in the office. For a posterior dislocation, the BoNT can be delivered to the PCA muscle with EMG guidance, thereby rebalancing toward the adductor muscle groups and moving the arytenoid anteriorly.[19]

13.13 Chronic Idiopathic Cough

Botulinum neurotoxin therapy has been used for the treatment of unexplained chronic cough syndromes with variable success. Cough is the fifth most common complaint in the primary care setting and cough lasting longer than 8 weeks is termed "chronic cough." Laryngeal etiologies for chronic cough may be the result of inflammation (acid, allergy, and asthma), irritation (chemical), mechanical trauma (chronic throat clearing), anatom-

ic factors (glottic stenosis, neoplasm, and vocal fold paralysis), or neurogenic inflammation along the respiratory tract. There are many idiopathic or poorly understood hyperspastic upper airway disorders described that share overlapping features; these disorders include neurogenic cough, irritable larynx syndrome, psychogenic cough, and unexplained chronic cough. BoNT injection may be considered when other diagnostic and treatment options have been exhausted and the larynx is believed to be the source of the cough, usually because of concomitant laryngeal dysfunction (laryngospasm, paresis, sensory neuropathy, dysphonia, or throat discomfort). The American College of Chest Physicians (ACCP) published a cough consensus panel report in 2006 which made specific recommendations of the workup and treatment for chronic cough in nonsmoking patients with clear chest radiography. We recommend that these guidelines be familiar to anyone considering treating patients with BoNT for chronic cough.[20]

There are several hypotheses of how Botox may be beneficial in chronic cough. In a neurogenic model of cough, there are numerous afferents carried via the sensory components of the vagus nerve that may become dysfunctional and sensitized, leading to a hyperexcitable state.[21] The BoNT may block the release of specific neuropeptides that are responsible for stimulating a pathogenic peripheral sensitization cycle. Alternatively, the Botox may also act simply as a "chemical splint" to help stop habituated behavior, reduce mechanical trauma elicited through vocal hyperfunction, and reestablish laryngeal homeostasis.

To date, there have been only small case series describing the use of BoNT in chronic cough. Sasieta et al reported the largest series of patients with refractory chronic cough treated with botulinum toxin A and reported treatment success (defined as over 50% reduction) in half of the 22 patients treated. Interestingly, the occurrence of liquid dysphagia after BoNT treatment had a positive predictive value of 84% and negative predictive value of 100% for treatment success, while development of dysphonia had no significant correlation with treatment outcomes.[22] In our experience, the use of BoNT for chronic cough has yielded more variable results. The BoNT may weaken the strength of the cough and decrease the traction and friction on the larynx, leading to a gradual decrease in traumatic inflammation. However, conversely, the patient may also experience increased aspiration and increased mucus, which may cause increased anxiety and provoke more cough and throat clearing. Concurrent pharmacologic treatment with antitussives is continued. The doses begin at about 2.5 U and continue for several treatment cycles at 2- to 3-month intervals.

13.14 Conclusion

Botulinum neurotoxin therapy is an extremely useful and versatile tool in the laryngologist's armamentarium. By chemically denervating the various laryngeal muscles, one is able to effectively diagnose and treat a number of disorders of the laryngopharynx. Most cases of dysphonia or dysphagia from a laryngeal cause are secondary to hyperfunctional behavior. Used as a "chemical knife," BoNT can allow for selective denervation of these hyperfunctional muscles, resulting in mitigation of symptoms and control of muscle spasm.

13.15 Key Points/Pearls

- Botulinum neurotoxin (BoNT) is a useful tool to denervate the laryngeal

musculature when symptoms of hyperfunction dominate the voice such as muscle tension dysphonia, vocal fold granuloma, tracheoesophageal puncture malfunction, puberphonia, tic disorders, and chronic cough.
- BoNT can also be used to selectively weaken targeted intrinsic laryngeal musculature to "rebalance" the vocal fold positioning in cases of bilateral vocal fold immobility, posterior glottic stenosis, and arytenoid dislocation or avulsion.
- BoNT is a titratable and useful tool typically reserved in cases of recalcitrant symptoms and serves as an additional option in the treatment regimen.

References

[1] Lin RJ, Klein-Fedyshin M, Rosen CA. Nimodipine improves vocal fold and facial motion recovery after injury: a systematic review and meta-analysis. Laryngoscope.; 129(4):943–951

[2] Ekbom DC, Garrett CG, Yung KC, et al. Botulinum toxin injections for new onset bilateral vocal fold motion impairment in adults. Laryngoscope.; 120(4):758–763

[3] Daniel SJ, Cardona I. Cricothyroid onabotulinum toxin A injection to avert tracheostomy in bilateral vocal fold paralysis. JAMA Otolaryngol Head Neck Surg.; 140(9):867–869

[4] Benninger MS, Hanick A, Hicks DM. Cricothyroid muscle botulinum toxin injection to improve airway for bilateral recurrent laryngeal nerve paralysis, a case series. J Voice.; 30(1):96–99

[5] Zealear DL, Billante CR, Courey MS, Sant'Anna GD, Netterville JL. Electrically stimulated glottal opening combined with adductor muscle Botox blockade restores both ventilation and voice in a patient with bilateral laryngeal paralysis. Ann Otol Rhinol Laryngol.; 111(6):500–506

[6] Blitzer A, Komisar A, Baredes S, Brin MF, Stewart C. Voice failure after tracheoesophageal puncture: management with botulinum toxin. Otolaryngol Head Neck Surg.; 113(6):668–670

[7] Pacheco PC, Karatayli-Ozgursoy S, Best S, Hillel A, Akst L. False vocal cord botulinum toxin injection for refractory muscle tension dysphonia: our experience with seven patients. Clin Otolaryngol.; 40(1):60–64

[8] Marras C, Andrews D, Sime E, Lang AE. Botulinum toxin for simple motor tics: a randomized, double-blind, controlled clinical trial. Neurology.; 56(5):605–610

[9] Kwak C, Jankovic J. Tics in Tourette syndrome and botulinum toxin. J Child Neurol.; 15(9):631–634

[10] Karkos PD, George M, Van Der Veen J, et al. Vocal process granulomas: a systematic review of treatment. Ann Otol Rhinol Laryngol.; 123(5):314–320

[11] Fink DS, Achkar J, Franco RA, Song PC. Interarytenoid botulinum toxin injection for recalcitrant vocal process granuloma. Laryngoscope.; 123(12):3084–3087

[12] Pham Q, Campbell R, Mattioni J, Sataloff R. Botulinum toxin injections into the lateral cricoarytenoid muscles for vocal process granuloma. J Voice.; 32(3):363–366

[13] Damrose EJ, Damrose JF. Botulinum toxin as adjunctive therapy in refractory laryngeal granuloma. J Laryngol Otol.; 122 (8):824–828

[14] Carroll TL, Gartner-Schmidt J, Statham MM, Rosen CA. Vocal process granuloma and glottal insufficiency: an overlooked etiology? Laryngoscope.; 120(1):114–120

[15] Hillel AT, Karatayli-Ozgursoy S, Samad I, et al. North American Airway Collaborative (NoAAC). Predictors of posterior glottic stenosis: a multi-institutional case-control study. Ann Otol Rhinol Laryngol.; 125(3):257–263

[16] Nathan CO, Yin S, Stucker FJ. Botulinum toxin: adjunctive treatment for posterior glottic synechiae. Laryngoscope.; 109(6):855–857

[17] Rontal E, Rontal M. Laryngeal rebalancing for the treatment of arytenoid dislocation. J Voice.; 12(3):383–388

[18] Rubin AD, Hawkshaw MJ, Sataloff RT. Vocal process avulsion. J Voice.; 19(4):702–706

[19] Rubin AD, Hawkshaw MJ, Moyer CA, Dean CM, Sataloff RT. Arytenoid cartilage dislocation: a 20-year experience. J Voice.; 19(4):687–701

[20] Irwin RS, Baumann MH, Bolser DC, et al. Diagnosis and management of cough executive summary: ACCP evidence-based clinical practice guidelines. Chest.; 129(1) Suppl: 1S–23S

[21] Altman KW, Irwin RS. Cough specialists collaborate for an interdisciplinary problem. Otolaryngol Clin North Am.; 43(1): xv–xix

[22] Sasieta HC, Iyer VN, Orbelo DM, et al. Bilateral thyroarytenoid botulinum toxin Type A injection for the treatment of refractory chronic cough. JAMA Otolaryngol Head Neck Surg.; 142 (9):881–888

14

Botulinum Neurotoxin for Migraine

Rachel Kaye, Jerome S. Schwartz, Brian E. Benson, and William J. Binder

Summary

Migraine is a leading cause of disability in the United States and worldwide. The socioeconomic burden of headache is significant and physicians are uniquely equipped to diagnose and treat headache disorders in order to ease patient suffering. A comprehensive history and physical examination allows the physician to categorize a patient's disorder and determine the risk of organic causes. Oral medications have variable efficacy and have an adverse-effect profile that may be unacceptable to patients. The management of headaches has evolved to include supplementary methods which can increase the number of patients who experience lasting reprieve from their affliction. Although its mechanism of action is incompletely understood, botulinum neurotoxin (BoNT) may offer relief from headache pain by acting on central and peripheral pathways. Adverse effects from BoNT are usually mild, transient, and often can be prevented by use of proper injection technique. Thus, BoNT chemodenervation is an adjunct therapy in managing migraine patients that is both effective and safe.

Keywords: migraine, headache, chemodenervation, botulinum toxin

14.1 Introduction

Headaches are one of the most common patient complaints when presenting to physicians; migraine plagues approximately 15% of adults and is listed as the second largest cause of disability worldwide as of 2016 review.[1] Migraine manifests as recurrent episodes of moderate to severe headache and can be accompanied by photophobia, phonophobia, and nausea. Additional symptoms include symptom waxing with physical exertion, unilateral localization, and pain of a throbbing character. The debilitating nature of these disorders can result in significant loss of productivity, reduced social engagement, and poorer quality of life. Other associated neuropsychiatric conditions such as depression and anxiety can complicate the morbidity of this disease. The socioeconomic burden can be measured in the billions of dollars incurred both direct (health care utilization) and indirect costs attributable to disability. Although the overwhelming majority of headache disorders are benign in nature, alternative organic etiologies (e.g., brain tumor or cerebral aneurysm) must be excluded.

14.2 Classification of Migraine

The International Headache Society (HIS) published a revised International Classification for Headache Disorders (ICHD-3) in 2018 which allows for a formal classification schema among practitioners.[2] Headache is characterized as primary or secondary and is differentiated from cranial neuropathies and other facial pain disorders. Primary headache denotes a disorder for which no identifiable structural or organic cause is known (e.g., migraine and tension headaches). Secondary headache is characterized by a known structural or systemic etiology. Furthermore, migraine can be subdivided based on the presence or absence of aura. Migraine without aura is the most prevalent subtype and may involve a higher frequency of attacks and greater disability than for those patients with aura. Migraine is further subdivided into chronic or episodic subtypes based on headache frequency. Chronic migraine represents 15 or more days of headache a month with 8 or more of those days with migraine headaches (▶ Table 14.1).

14.3 Etiology of Migraine

The pathophysiology of migraine disease is only partially understood despite ongoing research efforts. Current thinking suggests at least three mechanisms: extracranial arterial vasodilation, neurogenic inflammation, and decreased inhibition of central pain transmission. Cortical spreading depression, a phenomenon involving a slowly progressive wave of depolarization followed by electrical silence and hypoperfusion to the cerebral cortex, is thought to produce migraine aura and some believe that it represents an additional etiology of migraine headache.[3] Novel research using transcranial stimulation and biochemical analysis have provided convincing evidence that no single theory alone can yet explain the commencement, continuation, and resolution of migraine headaches, although several theories predominant current thinking.

Table 14.1 Diagnostic criteria for migraine

ICDH-3 code	Subtype	Definition/Characterization
1.1	Migraine without aura	• Recurrent (at least 5) headache attacks of 4–72 h in length • Two classic features (unilateral location, pulsating quality, moderate-severe pain, or aggravation with physical activity) • One associated symptom (nausea and/or vomiting or photophobia and phonophobia)
1.2	Migraine with aura	• One reversible aura symptom (visual, sensory, speech and/or language, motor, brainstem, retinal) • At least three characteristics (gradual spread over > 5 min, symptoms in succession, symptom lasts 5–60 min, unilateral symptom, positive symptom-scintillations or pins and needles, accompanied headache within 60 min)
1.3	Chronic migraine	• Headache > 15 d per month (8 d per month with migraine features) • Duration for > 3 mo
1.4	Complications of migraine	• Status migrainosus • Migrainous infarction • Persistent aura • Migraine aura-triggered seizure
1.5	Probable migraine	• Migraine-like attacks missing one criterion to fulfill above diagnoses
1.6	Episodic syndromes	• Recurrent gastrointestinal disturbance • Cyclic vomiting syndrome • Abdominal migraine • Benign paroxysmal vertigo • Benign paroxysmal torticollis

Source: Data from Headache Classification Committee of the International Headache Society (IHS). The International Classification of Headache Disorders 3rd ed. Cephalalgia 2018;38 (1):1–211.

The vasospasm-dilation theory describes changes in intra- and extracranial arterial diameter that promote migraine symptoms. Extracranial oligemia occurs during the headache's prodrome and continues into the early headache phase. Paradoxically, as the pain phase begins, vasodilation occurs with resultant persistent hyperemia. Directed efforts at promoting vasoconstriction resulted in trials with various antiplasma extravasation and vasoconstriction agents such as caffeine, serotonergic $5HT_{1B/1D}$ receptor agonists (triptans), and nonselective serotonergic agonists (ergot alkaloids) and met with variable success.

A dysfunction in the complex neurophysiologic system, the trigeminal neurovascular system, may also contribute to migraines. It is postulated that there are anatomic connections between the intracranial meninges and extracranial periosteum (and pericranial muscles).[4] This extracranial etiology for migraine headaches was initially proposed in the early 1950s and 1960s,[5,6] but has recently gained considerable support. Experiments in a mouse model showed an interconnected network of pain and sensory fibers traversing the calvarial bones through suture lines in young mice. These connections degenerated as the mice aged except at suture lines, where such connections remained intact.[7] Such sensory/pain fibers trifurcated, connecting the dura, the pia (by traversing the subarachnoid space), and the extracranial periosteum. Human studies have likewise found the persistence of sensory/pain fibers that traverse and connect the pericranial muscles, extracranial periosteum, cranial sutures, and the intracranial dura.[7,8,9] The presence and identification of this sensory/pain fiber network allows the theoretical construct where external pericranial irritation can lead to migraine headaches.

The presence of inflammation may modulate migraine severity; in patients with chronic migraine with bilateral occipital imploding headaches and associated chronic muscle tenderness, there was upregulation of inflammatory genes in human calvarial periosteum.[10] Some postulated that migraine headaches can originate in extracranial tissues that are hypersensitive to painful stimuli due to an inflammatory process. Further support for the theory of an extracranial source for migraines is shown through successful migraine reduction following nerve decompression surgeries,[11,12,13] occipital nerve stimulation,[14,15] and nerve blocks.[16,17] The theorized extracranial source for migraine headache has profound implications for the treatment and prophylaxis of this disorder.

14.4 Treatment Targets

A multitude of treatments have evolved, as many of the classic therapeutics have failed to effectively eliminate this disorder. Therapeutics aim to be abortive (halting progression and enacting resolution) or prophylactic (decrease attack frequency), but compliance remains low mostly due to perceived inadequate efficacy and/or adverse systemic effects. Of all the currently available treatments, only botulinum neurotoxin type A (BoNT-A) and topiramate have demonstrated efficacy in treating chronic migraine and received regulatory approval and BoNT is the only prophylactic treatment that is globally approved for chronic migraine.[18] Recently, calcitonin gene-related peptide (CGRP) receptor antagonists and monoclonal antibodies against the CGRP receptor sites have shown to be effective as a prophylactic treatment in chronic migraine. The duration of action is, however, reportedly to be limited to a 1-month period.[19]

Seminal reports on BoNT-A found that it was effective as a prophylactic medication but only for some patients.[20,21,22,23,24,25] In 2006, Jakubowski et al identified that the distinguishing factor for BoNT-A responders (>80% decrease in migraine days) was those with imploding or ocular headaches and boasted a 94 and 100% response rate, respectively. This was in contrast to those with exploding headaches who experienced only a 19% response rate.[26] Such a stratification could be explained if imploding and ocular headache development involved extracranial innervation which is suppressed by BoNT-A chemodenervation.

Although the exact mechanism of action of BoNT is much debated, one proposal includes inhibition of peripheral sensory neurons. BoNT inhibits the release of inflammatory mediators, specifically substance P,[27] CGRP,[28] and glutamate[29] by affecting their SNARE docking proteins. It is important to understand that although BoNT plays an important role in pain processing, it does not mediate acute pain. This is because A-delta or A-beta fibers are not mediated by neuropeptide release and therefore they are unaffected. Hence, BoNT can modulate pain processing without affecting the sensation of acute pain or resulting in local anesthesia upon injection.

Due to mounting evidence, BoNT-A injection has gained popularity as an alternative therapy for the treatment of migraine headache and was approved by the Food and Drug Administration (FDA) in 2010 as a prophylactic medication of chronic migraine. A 2018 Cochrane review reported that BoNT-A may reduce the number of migraine days for chronic migraine patients by 2 days per month. The same review called for further research with utility for episodic migraine as current results are inconclusive.[30]

14.5 Workup

A systematic and careful interview, examination, and documentation of symptoms can aid in obtaining the correct diagnosis for headache sufferers. A complete physical examination should be performed in order to determine the presence of cardiovascular, ophthalmologic, or neuromuscular etiologies or confounders. The ears, nose, throat, scalp, and neck should likewise be thoroughly examined. Specifically, secondary etiologies for headache should be sought and such physical exam investigations include attention to vital signs, emotional affect, cardiopulmonary evaluation, head and neck bruit auscultation, temporomandibular joint dysfunction, masses of the head and neck, and focal neurologic signs (visual field deficits, sensory deficits, asymmetric gait, papilledema, etc.).[31]

Characterization of the type of migraine headache will allow for patient education regarding expected results. As mentioned earlier, patients with imploding or ocular headaches have a much higher response rate (94 and 100%) compared to those with exploding headaches (19%).[26] This information is important in prognosticating the effectiveness of treatment benefit.

Neuroimaging must be part of the diagnostic workup by using either computed tomography or magnetic resonance imaging to exclude any secondary headache or organic disorder if clinical evidence suggests its presence. Lumbar puncture can be indicated in severe cases when one suspects subarachnoid hemorrhage, meningitis, severe alterations in cerebrospinal fluid (CSF) pressure, and/or meningeal carcinomatosis or lymphomatosis.[32] Although the prevalence of such pathology is low in headache sufferers, it is imperative that one maintains a high degree of suspicion to not overlook serious underlying pathology.

14.6 Anatomy

After a thorough history and examination, the anatomical subsites involved in the pain generation of headaches should be identified and documented for each patient. Typical injection sites in our experience can include glabella, temporal, frontal, suboccipital, and trapezius. Due to the large surface area usually affected by headaches, multiple injection sites are usually necessary. Practitioners vary widely in the number of injection sites and the total administered dose is often customized and ranges between 15 and 195 U reported in the literature. The standardized PREEMPT injection paradigm indicates a total dosage of 155 U distributed among 31 injection sites for fixed-site, fixed-dose injection paradigm, and up to 195 U distributed across 39 sites after adding the additional sites indicated in the follow-the-pain approach part of the paradigm.[33]

14.6.1 Forehead

The supratrochlear nerve is a branch of the frontal nerve which branches from the ophthalmic division of the trigeminal nerve. It enters the brow through the frontal notch/supratrochlear foramen then bifurcates within the retro-orbicularis oculi fat pad and then enters/pierces the corrugator supercilii and frontalis muscles to innervate the skin of the lower forehead in the midline. The corrugator supercilii muscle lies just above the supraorbital rim in an oblique direction angled toward the nasal dorsum. The supratrochlear nerve and vessels run alongside the medial extent of the corrugator, whereas the supraorbital bundle passes on its lateral aspect via the supraorbital foramen. The corrugator acts to depress the medial brow and usually produces vertical frown lines over the glabellar region. The procerus muscle is a triangular muscle that is continuous with the medial and inferior-most extent of the frontalis muscle. It inserts over the nasal bridge (attached to the glabellar skin) and acts as a medial brow depressor, thereby producing a horizontal frown line over the nasal bridge. The frontalis muscle is a large and broad muscle over the cranium of the forehead that extends from the supraorbital rim to the parietal region. Constriction (elicited during eyebrow elevation) creates horizontal forehead rhytids (▶ Fig. 14.1, ▶ Fig. 14.2).

14.6.2 Temporalis

The temporalis muscle is a fan-shaped muscle that covers the temporal region with its origination in the temporal line and insertion on the coronoid process of the mandible. The muscle can be identified by prompting the patient to clench their teeth as it is a muscle of mastication. It is innervated by the deep temporal nerves which are branches of the anterior division of the mandibular nerve (third division of the trigeminal nerve). The auriculotemporal nerve also supplies sensory fibers over the anterior temporal region (▶ Fig. 14.3, ▶ Fig. 14.4).

14.6.3 Posterior Scalp

Within the occipital region, the trapezius muscle, splenius capitis, and semispinalis muscles converge. The greater and lesser occipital nerves originate from the cervical plexus (branches of spinal nerve C2). The greater occipital nerve emerges below the suboccipital triangle, and crosses deep to the semispinalis capitis muscle to emerge above the superior nuchal line. It then pierces the scalp between the semispinalis capitis and trapezius muscles. The lesser occipital nerve curves around the posterior border of the sternocleidomastoid muscle and continues superiorly until it perforates

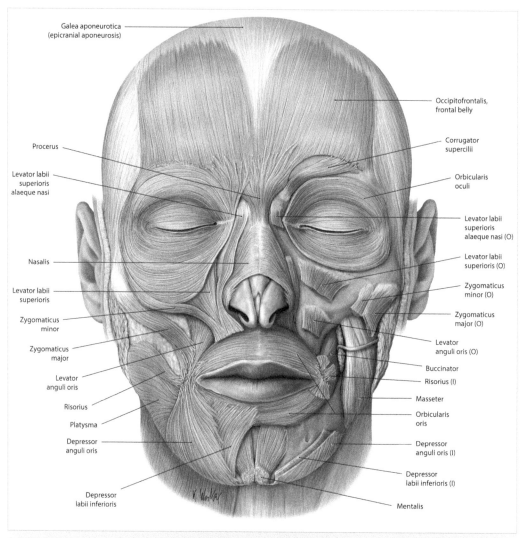

Galea aponeurotica
(epicranial aponeurosis)

Procerus

Levator labii
superioris
alaeque nasi

Nasalis

Levator labii
superioris

Zygomaticus
minor

Zygomaticus
major

Levator
anguli oris

Risorius

Platysma

Depressor
anguli oris

Depressor
labii inferioris

Occipitofrontalis,
frontal belly

Corrugator
supercilii

Orbicularis
oculi

Levator labii
superioris
alaeque nasi (O)

Levator labii
superioris (O)

Zygomaticus
minor (O)

Zygomaticus
major (O)

Levator
anguli oris (O)

Buccinator

Risorius (I)

Masseter

Orbicularis
oris

Depressor
anguli oris (I)

Depressor
labii inferioris (I)

Mentalis

Fig. 14.1 Glabellar and forehead injection sites. (From Gilroy AM et al. Atlas of Anatomy. 1st Ed. New York: Thieme Medical Publishers; 2008. Based on: Schuenke M, Schulte E, Schumacher U. THIEME Atlas of Anatomy: Head and Neuroanatomy. Illustrations by Voll M and Wesker K. 1st Ed. New York: Thieme Medical Publishers; 2008.)

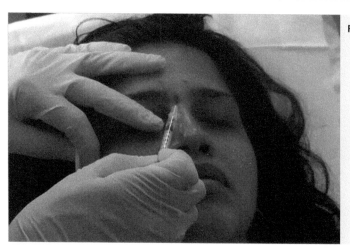

Fig. 14.2 Injection of the glabella.

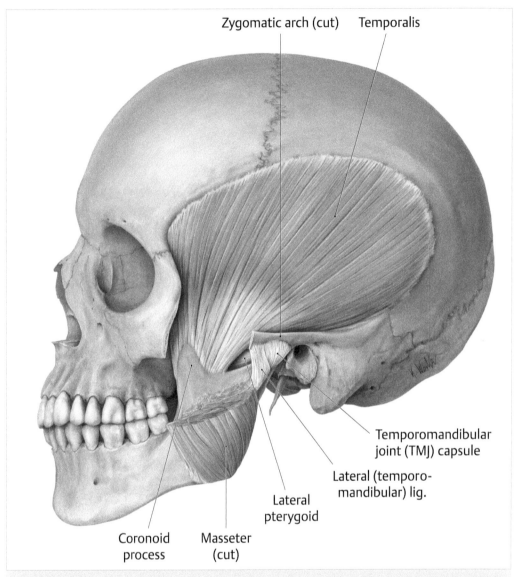

Zygomatic arch (cut)   Temporalis

Temporomandibular
joint (TMJ) capsule

Lateral (temporo-
mandibular) lig.

Lateral
pterygoid

Coronoid   Masseter
process   (cut)

Fig. 14.3 Temporal region injection sites. (From Gilroy AM et al. Atlas of Anatomy. 3rd Ed. New York: Thieme Medical Publishers; 2016. Based on: Schuenke M, Schulte E, Schumacher U. THIEME Atlas of Anatomy: Head and Neuroanatomy. Illustrations by Voll M and Wesker K. 1st Ed. New York: Thieme Medical Publishers; 2008.)

the deep fascia and innervating the post-auricular skin. The occipitalis muscle retracts the scalp backward and functions as a muscle complex with the frontalis muscle as they are linked by fascia (▶ Fig. 14.5).

14.7 Injection Technique

Currently, three formulations of BoNT-A (Botox, Dysport, and Xeomin) and one formulation of BoNT-B (Myobloc) are approved for clinical use and commercially

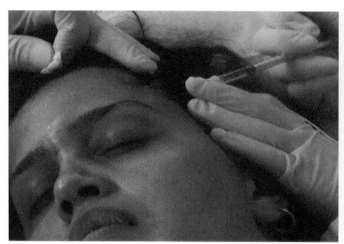

Fig. 14.4 Temporal injection.

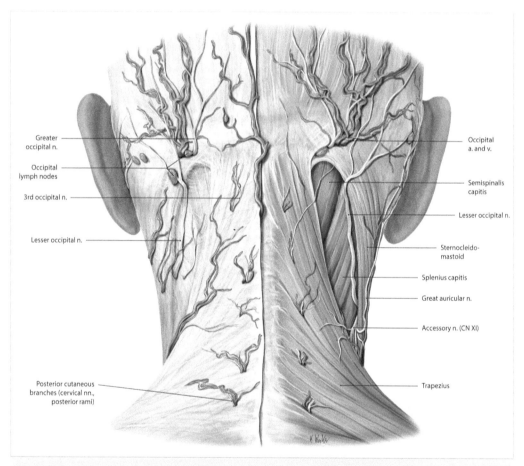

Fig. 14.5 Occipital and paraspinal injection sites. (From Gilroy AM et al. Atlas of Anatomy. 1st Ed. New York: Thieme Medical Publishers; 2008. Based on: Schuenke M, Schulte E, Schumacher U. THIEME Atlas of Anatomy: Head and Neuroanatomy. Illustrations by Voll M and Wesker K. 1st Ed. New York: Thieme Medical Publishers; 2008.)

available in the United States. These have varying dosing schedules and safety parameters and it is imperative that the practitioners have familiarity with each toxin formulation.

OnabotulinumtoxinA (Botox; Allergan plc, Irvine, CA) was the first type A toxin available in the United States. Each vial contains 50 or 100 units (U) of powdered BoNT-A, and requires dilution with 0.9% preservative-free saline. In our practice, we usually dilute each vial to a final concentration of 5.0 or 2.5 U per 0.1 mL stock. AbobotulinumtoxinA (Dysport, Galderma Laboratories, Fort Worth, TX) is available in 300 or 500 U vials, and incobotulinumtoxinA (Xeomin, Merz Pharmaceuticals, Raleigh, NC) is available in 50 and 100 U vials.

RimabotulinumtoxinB (Myobloc, Solstice Neurosciences LLC, Malvern, PA) is available in 2,500, 5,000, and 10,000 U vials all prediluted with 0.05% human serum albumin to a standard concentration of 500 U per 0.1 mL stock.

It is vital to note that BoNT is usually injected in an extramuscular plane and fascia, especially in the more medial occipital region and base of neck near the nuchal ridge. Furthermore, the injection sites can be mapped out to mirror the distribution of sensory nerves[33] based on the principles outlined in section "Etiology of Migraine." Two general techniques were described by PREEMPT and are used to determine injection sites: a fixed-dose technique or a customized follow-the-pain technique.[33]

Following the intended dilution (usually 4 mL/100 U of BoTN-A or 2.5 U per 0.1 mL) as mentioned earlier, the toxin is aspirated into a 1-mL syringe with an attached 30- or 32-gauge needle. Alternatively, if electromyographic (EMG) guidance is sought, a 27-gauge Teflon-coated hollow EMG needle is used. This can be helpful in directing injections near the deeper muscles of the temporal and occipital scalp. Sterile technique is used for toxin preparation and administration. The patient's skin is cleaned with alcohol to remove debris and contaminants. By limiting injections into the subcutaneous tissue or muscle belly, one reduces the risk of ecchymosis and injection-related tenderness.

14.7.1 Glabella and Frontalis Region

We follow the course of the supratrochlear nerve and supraorbital nerves (branches of the ophthalmic division of the trigeminal nerve). The injections are distributed centrally over the glabella and frontal areas of the forehead. They are injected at the nerve exit sites at the supratrochlear and supratrochlear foramina bilaterally and one site is injected centrally into the procerus muscle. The frontal region is injected by four to eight injection sites for each side in order to cover the entire central and lateral forehead areas. The BoNT will diffuse approximately 1 to 2 cm in diameter and into the frontalis muscle itself. It is important to counsel patients appropriately so that they can plan for frontalis muscle chemodenervation and resultant weakness of the forehead when attempting to raise their eyebrows. Similarly, it is important that injections of the forehead region should be performed symmetrically and using 0.1 to 0.2 mL volumes per injection site to avoid unwanted facial asymmetry.

14.7.2 Temporalis/Temple Region

When injecting the temporalis or temple region, there are four general areas of injection that align with the anterior, superior, inferior, and posterior quadrants of the temporalis muscle and treat the distribution of the auriculotemporal nerve anteriorly. In total, an average dose of 20 to 25 U of BoNT-A is used per side with an estimated 5 U per injection site.

14.7.3 Posterior Occipital and Postauricular Region of the Head

Posteriorly, the injections are above the nuchal ridge in the occipital and postauricular areas. The injections are distributed following the path of the greater and lesser occipital nerves as well as the occipitalis muscle and greater and lesser auricular nerves posterolaterally. The designated areas provide a greater latitude of injecting for the actual area of pain exhibited both extra- and intramuscularly instead of directed to a specific muscle path. Depending on the localization of pain, one to four sites are injected with 5 to 20 U per site. To target the occipital region, the needle point is directed just superior to the nuchal ridge and usually one to two injection sites are used with 5 to 7.5 U per site.

14.7.4 Posterior Neck

In the neck, BoNT can be injected into trigger points directed to the splenius capitis, paracervical muscles, as well as the trapezius muscles in tender areas usually localized below the nuchal ridge. One to four sites can be injected with an average of 5 to 20 U of BoNT-A per side.

14.8 Follow-up

Pain relief from BoNT chemodenervation may require several weeks to exhibit its maximal effect. Patients are therefore encouraged to maintain a headache diary both prior to and following injection to monitor its effect. Patients should make note to include any oral or supplementary medication that they take for breakthrough headache pain. Although the pharmacokinetic duration of the medication is approximately 12 weeks for BoNT-A, significant variability in clinical effect duration exists between patients possibly due to its neuromodulating effect and

relief for up to 56 weeks has been demonstrated.[34] Furthermore, similar to BoNT injections for other disorders, a patient's response to BoNT may change over time with some reporting greater therapeutic effect with repeat injections.[20] If patients do not receive an adequate response by 2 to 4 weeks following injection, they are asked to return to the office to consider a supplementary "booster" injection treatment. If the additional BoNT results in an improved response, then upon symptom recurrence the subsequent dosing will be an amalgam of the prior two doses.

14.9 Complications and Pitfalls

Adverse effects are usually mild and are by nature transient. They are usually due to inadvertent diffusion of BoNT to nearby structures. This diffusion can result in cosmetic challenges such as blepharoptosis, brow ptosis, and diplopia.[22] This can be prevented by taking care not to perform large volume (single site) injections, improper placement, or incorrect angle and direction of injection (i.e., direction of the needle near the brow should be directed superiorly).

Eyelid ptosis results from toxin diffusion through the superior aspect of the orbital septum, leading to chemodenervation and paralysis of the levator palpebrae superioris muscle. Injection at or inferior to the eyebrow near the midpupillary line increases the risk of ptosis. This can be prevented by using smaller injection volumes and injection placement at least 1 cm above the supraorbital rim at the midpupillary line. If ptosis occurs, then apraclonidine ophthalmic solution (alpha-2 adrenergic agonist) can be used to stimulate contraction of Muller's muscle to raise the eyelid 1 to 3 mm to reduce the severity of the ptosis until it naturally resolves with waning BoNT effect. However, apraclonidine cannot be used in patients with narrow angles or uncontrolled cardiovascular disease. Other sympathomimetic agents (e.g., brimonidine, phenylephrine, naphazoline) may have similar effects, although these are off-label usages.

Brow ptosis may develop from weakness of the inferolateral or supraorbital frontalis resulting in lateral or middle brow ptosis, respectively. Although injections are targeted at least 1 cm above the supraorbital rib, it is best to be prudent in patients with low-set brows. In these cases, it should be noted that only the upper part of the frontalis muscle should be injected, since the lower one-third of the muscle is primarily responsible for brow elevation. Partial chemodenervation is ideal in order to preserve some mobility of the frontalis muscle while obtaining migraine improvement. Additional brow elevation can be assisted by injecting BoNT into the surrounding depressors, including the ipsilateral superolateral orbicularis oculi muscle (lateral depressor), corrugator (medial depressor), or superomedial orbicularis oculi muscle (medial depressor).

Diplopia is an extremely rare complication when treating headache and is associated with lateral orbicularis oculi injections for hyperfunctional periorbital lines ("crow's feet"). This is due to toxin migration through the orbital septum and resulting in chemodenervation of the lateral rectus muscle. If injection is planned into the lateral orbicular region, it should be placed superficially (subcutaneously) at approximately 1 cm lateral to the lateral orbital rim (or 1.5 cm lateral to the lateral canthus). Diplopia warrants an immediate referral to ophthalmology for optimization.

Additional minor sequelae occur due to the delivery process of injection, such as local pain, erythema, edema, ecchymosis, and short-term hypoesthesia. Application of ice prior or following intramuscular injections can reduce the incidence of pain, edema, and erythema. Vessel disruption is prevented by having patients avoid aspirin, nonsteroidal anti-inflammatory drugs (NSAIDs), and vitamin E for 7 days prior to injection, and by avoidance of small vessels through visual confirmation and avoidance of larger caliber vessels by palpation. Local pain and tenderness can be further minimized by slowly infusing the injection with a small-gauge needle (30 or 32 gauge) and by taking care to avoid periosteum, as this is not only an unnecessary depth of injection but also painful.

14.10 Key Points/Pearls

- Botulinum neurotoxin (BoNT) chemodenervation boasts advantages beyond simple neuromuscular blockade.
- BoNT has utility in myofascial and inflammatory syndromes, such as chronic migraine.
- Patients who were previously recalcitrant to treatment with oral medications may be responsive to BoNT and may experience significant relief.
- BoNT is posited to have both central and peripheral mechanisms of action by affecting neuromodulation of nociception and inflammatory signal cascades:
  - The exact mechanism of action remains elusive along with the pathophysiology for migraine generation itself.
  - Further research efforts are required to advance our current understanding of these processes.
- The adverse effects of BoNT are infrequent, usually mild, and by definition temporary.
- BoNT represents a safe alternative therapy for treating migraine and headache symptoms.

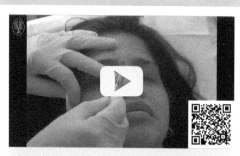

Video 14.1 Migraine. In this patient with left temporal and postocular pain, the area of the glabella (supraorbital and supratrochlear nerves) is injected in three places with 2.5 U/0.1 mL at each point as shown. The left anterior temporalis muscle is also injected with 2.5 U/0.1 mL of Botox in three to five different sites. [1:24]

References

[1] Disease GBD, Injury I, Prevalence C, GBD 2016 Disease and Injury Incidence and Prevalence Collaborators. Global, regional, and national incidence, prevalence, and years lived with disability for 328 diseases and injuries for 195 countries, 1990–2016: a systematic analysis for the Global Burden of Disease Study 2016. Lancet.; 390(10100):1211–1259

[2] Headache Classification Committee of the International Headache Society (IHS), . The International Classification of Headache Disorders. 3rd ed. Cephalalgia.; 38(1):1–211

[3] Bolay H, Reuter U, Dunn AK, Huang Z, Boas DA, Moskowitz MA. Intrinsic brain activity triggers trigeminal meningeal afferents in a migraine model. Nat Med.; 8(2):136–142

[4] Burstein R, Blake P, Schain A, Perry C. Extracranial origin of headache. Curr Opin Neurol.; 30(3):263–271

[5] Wolff HG, Tunis MM, Goodell H. Studies on headache; evidence of damage and changes in pain sensitivity in subjects with vascular headaches of the migraine type. AMA Arch Intern Med.; 92(4):478–484

[6] Selby G, Lance JW. Observations on 500 cases of migraine and allied vascular headache. J Neurol Neurosurg Psychiatry.; 23:23–32

[7] Kosaras B, Jakubowski M, Kainz V, Burstein R. Sensory innervation of the calvarial bones of the mouse. J Comp Neurol.; 515(3):331–348

[8] Schueler M, Messlinger K, Dux M, Neuhuber WL, De Col R. Extracranial projections of meningeal afferents and their impact on meningeal nociception and headache. Pain.; 154(9): 1622–1631

[9] Schueler M, Neuhuber WL, De Col R, Messlinger K. Innervation of rat and human dura mater and pericranial tissues in the parieto-temporal region by meningeal afferents. Headache.; 54(6):996–1009

[10] Perry CJ, Blake P, Buettner C, et al. Upregulation of inflammatory gene transcripts in periosteum of chronic migraineurs: Implications for extracranial origin of headache. Ann Neurol.; 79(6):1000–1013

[11] Janis JE, Barker JC, Javadi C, Ducic I, Hagan R, Guyuron B. A review of current evidence in the surgical treatment of migraine headaches. Plast Reconstr Surg.; 134(4) Suppl 2:131S–141S

[12] Chepla KJ, Oh E, Guyuron B. Clinical outcomes following supraorbital foraminotomy for treatment of frontal migraine headache. Plast Reconstr Surg.; 129(4):656e–662e

[13] Guyuron B, Reed D, Kriegler JS, Davis J, Pashmini N, Amini S. A placebo-controlled surgical trial of the treatment of migraine headaches. Plast Reconstr Surg.; 124(2):461–468

[14] Saper JR, Dodick DW, Silberstein SD, McCarville S, Sun M, Goadsby PJ, ONSTIM Investigators. Occipital nerve stimulation for the treatment of intractable chronic migraine headache: ONSTIM feasibility study. Cephalalgia.; 31(3):271–285

[15] Young WB. Occipital nerve stimulation for chronic migraine. Curr Pain Headache Rep.; 18(2):396

[16] Dach F, Éckeli AL, Ferreira KdosS, Speciali JG. Nerve block for the treatment of headaches and cranial neuralgias - a practical approach. Headache.; 55 Suppl 1:59–71

[17] Blumenfeld A, Ashkenazi A, Evans RW. Occipital and trigeminal nerve blocks for migraine. Headache.; 55(5):682–689

[18] Aurora SK, Brin MF. Chronic migraine: an update on physiology, imaging, and the mechanism of action of two available pharmacologic therapies. Headache.; 57(1):109–125

[19] Tso AR, Goadsby PJ. Anti-CGRP monoclonal antibodies: the next era of migraine prevention. Curr Treat Options Neurol.; 19(8):27

[20] Binder WJ, Brin MF, Blitzer A, Schoenrock LD, Pogoda JM. Botulinum toxin type A (BOTOX) for treatment of migraine headaches: an open-label study. Otolaryngol Head Neck Surg.; 123(6):669–676

[21] Ondo WG, Vuong KD, Derman HS. Botulinum toxin A for chronic daily headache: a randomized, placebo-controlled, parallel design study. Cephalalgia.; 24(1):60–65

[22] Silberstein S, Mathew N, Saper J, Jenkins S, For the BOTOX Migraine Clinical Research Group. Botulinum toxin type A as a migraine preventive treatment. Headache.; 40(6):445–450

[23] Tepper SJ, Bigal ME, Sheftell FD, Rapoport AM. Botulinum neurotoxin type A in the preventive treatment of refractory headache: a review of 100 consecutive cases. Headache.; 44 (8):794–800

[24] Dodick DW, Mauskop A, Elkind AH, DeGryse R, Brin MF, Silberstein SD, BOTOX CDH Study Group. Botulinum toxin type A for the prophylaxis of chronic daily headache: subgroup analysis of patients not receiving other prophylactic medications: a randomized double-blind, placebo-controlled study. Headache.; 45(4):315–324

[25] Evers S, Vollmer-Haase J, Schwaag S, Rahmann A, Husstedt IW, Frese A. Botulinum toxin A in the prophylactic treatment of migraine–a randomized, double-blind, placebo-controlled study. Cephalalgia.; 24(10):838–843

[26] Jakubowski M, McAllister PJ, Bajwa ZH, Ward TN, Smith P, Burstein R. Exploding vs. imploding headache in migraine prophylaxis with Botulinum Toxin A. Pain.; 125(3):286–295

[27] Welch MJ, Purkiss JR, Foster KA. Sensitivity of embryonic rat dorsal root ganglia neurons to Clostridium botulinum neurotoxins. Toxicon.; 38(2):245–258

[28] Durham PL, Cady R, Cady R. Regulation of calcitonin gene-related peptide secretion from trigeminal nerve cells by botulinum toxin type A: implications for migraine therapy. Headache.; 44(1):35–42, discussion 42–43

[29] Cui M, Khanijou S, Rubino J, Aoki KR. Subcutaneous administration of botulinum toxin A reduces formalin-induced pain. Pain.; 107(1–2):125–133

[30] Herd CP, Tomlinson CL, Rick C, et al. Botulinum toxins for the prevention of migraine in adults. Cochrane Database Syst Rev.; 6:CD011616

[31] Taylor FR. Diagnosis and classification of headache. Prim Care.; 31(2):243–259, v

[32] Evans RW. Diagnostic testing for headache. Med Clin North Am.; 85(4):865–885

[33] Blumenfeld AM, Silberstein SD, Dodick DW, Aurora SK, Brin MF, Binder WJ. Insights into the functional anatomy behind the PREEMPT injection paradigm: guidance on achieving optimal outcomes. Headache.; 57(5):766–777

[34] Aurora SK, Winner P, Freeman MC, et al. Onabotulinumtoxin-A for treatment of chronic migraine: pooled analyses of the 56-week PREEMPT clinical program. Headache.; 51(9):1358–1373

15
Botulinum Neurotoxin for Chronic Tension Headache

Nwanmegha Young and Brian E. Benson

Summary

Headache is one of the most common complaints of individuals seeking medical help. Clinical symptomatology is used to differentiate between two categories of headaches: tension-type headache and migraine headache. While tension-type headaches affect a majority of adults at some point in their lives, chronic tension-type headaches affect a minority of headache sufferers. High-level evidence supports the use of botulinum toxin for the treatment of chronic daily migraine, but there is a lack of evidence supporting the efficacy of botulinum toxin for chronic tension-type headache. However, due to the symptom crossover between tension-type headaches and migraine, botulinum toxin can be considered in those patients who fail standard therapies.

Keywords: headache, tension-type headache, muscle tension headache, botulinum neurotoxin

15.1 Introduction

Tension-type headache or TTH is the most common form of headache. It is sometimes referred to as "stress headache" or "muscle tension headache." There are two classifications of TTH: episodic tension-type headache (ETTH), which occurs randomly and infrequently, and chronic tension-type headache (CTTH), which occurs daily or continuously on at least 15 days per month, although the intensity of the pain may vary during a 24-hour cycle.[1] It is estimated that 30 to 80% of the adult population in the United States suffer from occasional TTH, yet only 3% suffer from CTTH.[2]

Symptoms of TTH include a tight feeling in head or neck muscles or a tightening band-like sensation around the neck or head, which creates a "vise-like" ache. The pain is typically found in the forehead, temples, or the back of the head or neck. However, there is frequently significant crossover between the symptoms of TTH and migraine without aura. In fact, in the Spectrum study, 71% of the participants initially diagnosed with episodic TTH subsequently had their diagnosis changed to migraine or migrainous headache after their headache diary was reviewed by the investigators.[3] However, the hallmark feature of TTH is increased pericranial tenderness. The third edition of the International Classification of Headache Disorders (ICHD-III) subdivides TTH into four divisions: infrequent episodic, frequent episodic, chronic, and probable; see ▶ Table 15.1 and ▶ Table 15.2.[4]

Table 15.1 Tension-type headache (episodic form): general diagnostic criteria (B–E)

Data from International Headache Society.
The International Classification of Headache Disorders 3rd Ed (ICHD-3). Cephalalgia 2018;38(1):1–211

B. Headache lasting from 30 min to 7 d

C. At least two of the following pain characteristics:

1. Bilateral location
2. Pressing or tightening (nonpulsating) quality
3. Mild or moderate intensity
4. Not aggravated by routine physical activity, such as walking or climbing stairs

D. Both of the following:

1. No nausea or vomiting (anorexia can occur)
2. No more than either photophobia or phonophobia

E. Not better accounted for by another ICH-3 diagnosis

Table 15.2 Tension-type headache: specific diagnostic criteria

Data from International Headache Society.
The International Classification of Headache Disorders 3rd Ed (ICHD-3). Cephalalgia 2018;38(1):1–211

2.1. Infrequent episodic tension-type headache

A. At least 10 episodes that occur on less than 1 d/mo (< 12 d/y) that fulfill criteria B–D

2.2. Frequent episodic tension-type headache

A. At least 10 episodes that occur on 1–14 d/mo on average for more than 3 mo which fulfill criteria B–D

2.3. Chronic tension-type headache

A. Headache that occurs on 15 or more days per month, on average for more than 3 mo (180 or more days per year), which fulfills criteria B–D

B. Headache that lasts hours or may be continuous

1. At least two of the following four characteristics:
   - Bilateral location
   - Pressing or tightening (nonpulsating) quality
   - Mild or moderate intensity
   - Not aggravated by routine physical activity such as walking or climbing stairs
2. Both of the following:
   - No more than photophobia, phonophobia, or mild nausea
   - Neither moderate or severe nausea nor vomiting
3. Not better accounted for by another ICHD-3 diagnosis

2.4. Probable tension-type headache

A. Tension-type headache missing one of the features required to fulfill all criteria for a type or subtype of tension-type headache coded above, and not fulfilling criteria for another headache disorder

The new fourth category of "probable" TTH was created due to the difficulty differentiating between TTH and migraine without aura. The etiology of TTH is thought to be related to cervical myofascial activity involving the neck, face, and scalp, which likely reflects a complex syndrome involving peripheral nociceptors in ETTH and central dysnociception in CTTH.[1]

Nonpharmacologic treatments such as relaxation and electromyography (EMG) biofeedback therapies, cognitive behavioral interventions, and various physical therapy techniques have shown various degrees of success at reducing the frequency and severity of TTH. Medications used to treat chronic daily headache include simple analgesics, such as aspirin and paracetamol, and nonsteroidal anti-inflammatory drugs (NSAIDs), such as ibuprofen and naproxen sodium. The addition of caffeine increases the efficacy of these medications. Prophylactic medications such as tricyclic antidepressants, selective serotonin reuptake inhibitors (SSRIs), the antispasmodic drug tizanidine, and topiramate may provide additional relief for some patients. Unfortunately, current pharmacotherapy for CTTH can be limited by either incomplete efficacy or intolerable side effects.

Given its effects on nociception and muscle contraction, botulinum neurotoxin (BoNT) appears to be an attractive agent in the prophylaxis of TTH. In addition to its well-known effects in reducing muscle contractions, it may also block the release of pain mediators such as substance P, glutamate, and calcitonin gene-related peptide.[5] Our experience with temporomandibular disorder (TMD) patients with TTH shows a 70% response rate (where a response is a 50% or greater reduction in intensity or frequency of headache) in an open-label study. Early, nonrandomized series provided encouraging data supporting the role of prophylactic treatment with BoNT-A.[6] The results of the PREEMPT (Phase 3 REsearch Evaluating Migraine Prophylaxis Therapy) trials 1 and 2 strongly supported the use of BoNT-A for chronic migraine prophylaxis.[7,8] Given the significant crossover between the symptoms of TTH and migraine, a plausible mechanism for BoNT-A prophylaxis of TTH was established. In contrast, the results of more recent, randomized, controlled trials in 2004 for the efficacy of BoNT in the prophylactic treatment of TTH are negative.[9,10] Meta-analysis in 2012 likewise revealed no association with reduction in number of TTH.[11,12] However, those findings do not rule out a possible role of BoNT-A in patients with severe, unremitting forms of CTTH, especially those like the following:

- Patients who have failed to respond adequately to conventional treatments.
- Patients with unacceptable side effects from existing treatment.
- Patients in whom standard preventive treatments are contraindicated.
- Patients who are misusing, overusing, or abusing medications.
- Patients with spasm or trigger points involving the jaw or head.

15.2 Workup

The diagnosis of TTH is based on a comprehensive history and neurologic examination, frequently in conjunction with a headache diary, and imaging studies. The diagnostic criteria for TTH are listed in ▶ Table 15.1 and ▶ Table 15.2.

15.3 Anatomy

The pertinent anatomy is reviewed in Chapter 14.

15.4 Injection Technique

There are no formal clinical guidelines for the use of BoNT in the treatment of headaches. Based on our experience, we typically employ one of two typical approaches to injecting BoNT to relieve headache pain. The "fixed-site" approach is typically employed in patients with migraine features, whereas the "follow-the-pain" approach is typically used for patients with TTHs. Both approaches can be combined for patients with features of mixed headache.

15.4.1 Fixed-Site Approach

Botulinum neurotoxin type A is injected into the procerus (5 units [U], one site), corrugator (2.5 U each, two sites [medial and lateral]), frontalis (2.5 U each, five sites on each side), and temporalis (2.5 U each, four sites on each side) muscles. Although "blind" injection technique may be used, we find that EMG guidance is useful to help target the appropriate muscles, especially the thin temporalis muscle.

15.4.2 Follow-the-Pain Approach

Using EMG guidance, BoNT-A is injected into the frontalis (2.5 U each, five sites on each side), temporalis (2.5 U each, four sites on each side), occipitalis (2.5–5 U on each side), trapezius (7.5–15 U on each side), semispinalis capitis (7.5–15 U on each side), and/or splenius capitis muscles, as deemed appropriate.

15.5 Follow-up

If effective, injections are typically repeated every 3 to 4 months, as necessary.

15.6 Complications

Ptosis of the eyelid and the eyebrow has been reported in less than 2% of patients. Other reported potential complications include neck weakness, bruising, and flulike symptoms.

15.7 Conclusion

Clinical and preclinical studies performed to date suggest that BoNT-A may work at multiple points in the pathophysiologic cascade of headache, although it is not yet clear which of these points are quantitatively most important. Although the efficacy of BoNT-A to ameliorate the symptoms of chronic migraine has been established, further studies need to be performed to determine which, if any, TTH patients will most benefit from BoNT injection.

15.8 Key Points/Pearls

- The hallmark feature of tension-type headache (TTH) is pericranial tenderness.
- A new "probable" category has been added to the definition of TTH.

Chronic Tension Headaches

Most chronic tension headaches are related to a "vise-like" pain across the head. We start with injections of the temporalis muscles bilaterally, as can be seen in **Video 12.1**. We also usually inject across the forehead, as outlined in **Video 9.2**, on glabellar frown lines. Occasionally, patients also have pain in the occiput or along the nuchal lines; these injections can be seen as part of **Video 7.1** on cervical dystonia.

References

[1] Fumal A, Schoenen J. Tension-type headache: current research and clinical management. Lancet Neurol.; 7(1):70–83

[2] Rasmussen BK, Jensen R, Schroll M, Olesen J. Epidemiology of headache in a general population–a prevalence study. J Clin Epidemiol.; 44(11):1147–1157

[3] Lipton RB, Cady RK, Stewart WF, Wilks K, Hall C. Diagnostic lessons from the spectrum study. Neurology.; 58(9) Suppl 6: S27–S31

[4] International Headache Society. The International Classification of Headache Disorders, 3rd ed (ICHD-III). Cephalalgia.; 38(1):1–211

[5] Aoki KR. Pharmacology of botulinum neurotoxin. Otolaryngol Head Neck Surg.; 15:81–85

[6] Blumenfeld A. Botulinum toxin type A as an effective prophylactic treatment in primary headache disorders. Headache.; 43(8):853–860

[7] Aurora SK, Dodick DW, Turkel CC, et al. PREEMPT 1 Chronic Migraine Study Group. OnabotulinumtoxinA for treatment of chronic migraine: results from the double-blind, randomized, placebo-controlled phase of the PREEMPT 1 trial. Cephalalgia.; 30(7):793–803

[8] Diener HC, Dodick DW, Aurora SK, et al. PREEMPT 2 Chronic Migraine Study Group. OnabotulinumtoxinA for treatment of chronic migraine: results from the double-blind, randomized, placebo-controlled phase of the PREEMPT 2 trial. Cephalalgia.; 30(7):804–814

[9] Padberg M, de Bruijn SF, de Haan RJ, Tavy DL. Treatment of chronic tension-type headache with botulinum toxin: a double-blind, placebo-controlled clinical trial. Cephalalgia.; 24 (8):675–680

[10] Schulte-Mattler WJ, Krack P, BoNTTH Study Group. Treatment of chronic tension-type headache with botulinum toxin A: a randomized, double-blind, placebo-controlled multicenter study. Pain.; 109(1–2):110–114

[11] Jackson JL, Kuriyama A, Hayashino Y. Botulinum toxin A for prophylactic treatment of migraine and tension headaches in adults: a meta-analysis. JAMA.; 307(16):1736–1745

[12] Wieckiewicz M, Grychowska N, Zietek M, Wieckiewicz G, Smardz J. Evidence to use botulinum toxin injections in tension-type headache management: a systematic review. Toxins (Basel).; 9(11):E370

16
Botulinum Neurotoxin for Trigeminal Neuralgia

Elizabeth Guardiani, Andrew Blitzer, Lesley French Childs, and Ronda E. Alexander

Summary

Trigeminal neuralgia (TN) is a unilateral facial pain disorder characterized by brief, paroxysmal, sharp lancinating pains that are recurrent and limited to the distribution of one or more divisions of the trigeminal nerve. The pain attacks are typically precipitated by innocuous cutaneous stimuli within specific "trigger zones" and may or may not be accompanied by persistent facial pain in the same distribution. Nerve damage, often from vascular compression, leads to chronic persistent facial pain due to peripheral and central sensitization to nociceptive stimuli. First-line treatment is with anticonsultants such as carbamazepine with more invasive procedures, such as microvascular decompression and stereotactic radiosurgery, reserved for refractory cases. Botulinum toxin A (BoNT-A) injections offer a safe and effective alternative to traditional therapies. Intradermal injections of BoNT-A are performed in 2.5-unit aliquots per square centimeter in the affected area of the face. The most common side effects are facial asymmetry and local injection site reaction.

Keywords: trigeminal neuralgia, facial pain, botulinum toxin, trigeminal neuropathy

16.1 Introduction

Trigeminal neuralgia (TN), as defined by the International Association for the Study of Pain (IASP), is a unilateral facial pain disorder that is characterized by brief, paroxysmal, sharp lancinating pains that are recurrent, and limited to the distribution of one or more divisions of the trigeminal nerve.[1] The prevalence of this disorder is approximately 1 in 25,000, and it is slightly more common in women than in men. It also affects middle-aged or older people more frequently.[2]

In the latest classification of the International Headache Society, TN was divided into two distinct groups: classical TN and painful trigeminal neuropathy. Classical TN includes idiopathic cases in addition to those with vascular compression of the fifth cranial nerve; painful trigeminal neuropathy is diagnosed in cases where there is damage to the trigeminal nerve from another disorder, including herpes zoster, multiple sclerosis, trauma, and space occupying lesions, resulting in facial pain.[3] Classical TN can be further divided into purely paroxysmal or with concomitant persistent facial pain, with the paroxysmal variant being more common and amenable to treatment. The pain attacks are typically precipitated by innocuous cutaneous stimuli within specific "trigger zones," but can also be spontaneous (although precipitated attacks are required for diagnosis). The attacks can leave some patients unable to eat, drink, brush their teeth, or shave. Attacks typically last a few seconds to 2 minutes, but can be more prolonged and severe as time goes on.

The peripheral neuropathic process is a result of damage to the trigeminal nerve, resulting in irritation and accumulation of nociceptive agents. The accumulation of pain modulators along with focal inflammation lowers the sensory threshold of peripheral nerve endings to nociceptive stimuli. Then peripheral sensitization increases arrival of the nociceptive signals into the spinal cord and sensitizes the sensory spinal cord neurons, leading to chronic pain.[4]

Nerve damage can result from demyelination of the sensory fibers within the proximal nerve root of the trigeminal nerve.[5] Most cases of classical TN (80–90%) have an overlying blood vessel causing compression at the root entry zone. The offending vessel can be the superior cerebellar artery (75%), the anterior inferior cerebellar artery (10%), or a vein.[6] Focal demyelination within or near this area has been documented on histologic examination of specimens taken during microvascular decompression in the immediate vicinity of the indentation, with the demyelinated axons found to be in direct apposition.[7] The A-δ thinly myelinated nociceptive fibers may be particularly vulnerable to such changes.[8] This pathologic arrangement may lead to abnormal nonsynaptic ephaptic transmission to adjacent fibers.[9] Moreover, because fibers for light touch and pain are closest in proximity within the root entry zone, this theory provides a ready explanation for the paroxysmal pain provoked by cutaneous stimuli.[5]

Many approaches have been employed to alleviate the pain and reduce the frequency of pain attacks in this disorder. Pharmacotherapy with anticonvulsive drugs remains the first-line therapy, in particular carbamazepine or oxcarbazepine. In patients with TN refractory to medical therapy, microvascular decompression, percutaneous approaches to the Gasserian ganglion, and stereotactic radiotherapy may also be considered, depending on surgeon experience and patient preference; however, these procedures carry additional morbidity.[10]

Botulinum neurotoxin type A (BoNT-A) has been successfully utilized to several pain syndromes including migraine and occipital neuralgia as discussed in previous chapters in this book. The mechanism by which BoNT-A influences pain has been described through a number of in vitro and in vivo studies. In vitro, investigators have demonstrated that application of BoNT-A to cultured sensory neurons inhibits the release of calcitonin gene-related peptide (CGRP), glutamate, and other pain transmitters after cleaving the SNARE proteins. In animal studies, toxin has been demonstrated to travel to the spinal cord and inhibits the release of substance P from spinal neurons along with a reduction of c-Fos expression at the spinal cord level.[11] The peripheral injection of BoNT prior to the application of a noxious stimuli has also been shown to reduce local accumulation of pain transmitters such as glutamate as well as improve behavioral manifestations of pain in an animal model.[11,12]

These findings led to the application of BoNT-A in the treatment of classical TN as well as painful trigeminal neuropathy. In recent years, BoNT-A has gained popularity in treating patients with TN that is refractory to medical and occasionally surgical treatment given its low side-effect profile.[13,14,15,16] BoNT-A has been shown to have significant benefit when compared with placebo in the reduction of paroxysmal attacks and visual analog scale (VAS) scores for pain in patients with classical TN as well as reduce VAS scores in patients with postherpetic painful trigeminal neuropathy.[4,17] A recent review found that there is level A evidence (effective) for BoNT therapy in TN, with three double-blind and one prospective single-blind clinical trials having assessed the efficacy of BoNT treatment in TN.[18]

16.2 Workup and Patient Selection

The diagnostic workup for patients amenable to BoNT-A treatment should elicit a history of pain that has become resistant to pharmacotherapy, or intolerance to the side effects of the medications. These patients had been previously labeled surgical candidates; however, BoNT-A treatment offers a less invasive option for pain alleviation with good results and minimal side effects.

The history should definitively rule out other causes of facial pain. Because of the association with multiple sclerosis, patients should be asked about neurologic symptoms (e.g., dizziness, focal weakness, ataxia, vision changes) and other atypical symptoms that might lead to another diagnosis.

The physician should perform a careful head and neck examination, with emphasis on the neurologic aspect. An otologic, oral, and temporomandibular joint (TMJ) examination should be done to search for other causes of facial pain. TN patients usually have a normal neurologic examination, and the finding of trigger points nearly confirms the diagnosis.[19] Documentation of facial nerve function and facial symmetry prior to the injections must be emphasized in the neurologic head and neck examination. Magnetic resonance imaging (MRI) of the brain should be performed for all patients presenting with TN, if one has not yet been performed prior to presentation.[10]

Absolute contraindications to BoNT use include a known allergy or sensitivity to the toxin, and diseases that might interfere with neuromuscular transmission, such as myasthenia gravis, Lambert-Eaton syndrome, amyotrophic lateral sclerosis, and others. BoNT should not be used in pregnant or lactating women or in patients taking aminoglycosides, as these can interfere with neuromuscular transmission.

16.3 Injection Technique

The identification and treatment of trigger zones on the face will provide the most benefit to the patient. At each visit, it is useful to draw a grid on the patient's face in the region of allodynia or hyperesthesia (▶ Fig. 16.1). Next, 2.5 unit (U)/ 0.1 mL intradermal injections of BoNT per square centimeter are administered within the grid (▶ Fig. 16.2). Careful record keeping using a facial map or diagram facilitates administering repeat injections as necessary, although the region of sensitivity is likely to change at each visit. The amount of toxin to be injected is tailored to the individual. Wide variations have been published in the literature, with one case report documenting the administration of 100 U to a single trigger site.[3]

16.4 Follow-up

Frequency of administration also needs to be individualized. Duration of effect in the literature ranges from weeks to

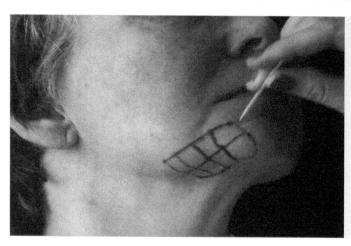

Fig. 16.1 Grid drawn on region of hyperesthesia/allodynia.

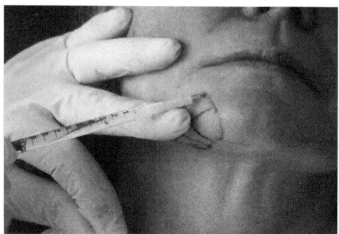

Fig. 16.2 Intradermal injection at the intersection of grid lines.

6 months. Initial treatments should be accompanied by a pain diary, which enables the patient and physician to track the waning and waxing of symptoms with treatment.

16.5 Complications and Pitfalls

Side effects of BoNT injections are generally a result of its effect on motor synapses, including the possibility of facial weakness and asymmetry after treatment. Contralateral injections can be performed if desired to improve facial symmetry. Facial edema, erythema, and hypoesthesia of the treated regions have also been reported.[13,17]

16.6 Conclusion

Botulinum neurotoxin treatment of TN represents a safe and effective treatment modality. Further studies will help clarify ideal injection schedules and approaches.

16.7 Key Points/Pearls

- Trigeminal neuralgia (TN) is unilateral facial pain disorder that is characterized by brief, paroxysmal, sharp lancinating pains that are recurrent, and limited to the distribution of one or more divisions of the trigeminal nerve.
- Botulinum neurotoxin type A (BoNT-A) has sensory effects as well as motor

effects and can be used for certain pain disorders

- BoNT-A can be used as an alternative or adjunct to oral medications for TN.
- When using BoNT-A for the treatment of TN, a grid is made on the patient's face in the distribution of symptoms and BoNT-A is injected in 2.5 U aliquots per square centimeter. The dose can be adjusted as needed in subsequent injections.

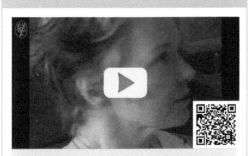

Video 16.1 Trigeminal neuralgia, midface. Initially, a toothpick is used to help map areas of allodynia and hyperesthesia. A 1-cm grid is created of the area. Then, 2.5 U/0.1 mL of Botox is injected intradermally at each intersecting point. [2:47]

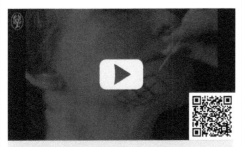

Video 16.2 Trigeminal neuralgia, lower face. [0:19]

References

[1] Merskey H, Bogduk N. Classification of Chronic Pain: Descriptions of Chronic Pain Syndromes and Definitions of Pain Terms. Seattle: IASP Press; 1994:59–71

[2] Katusic S, Williams DB, Beard CM, Bergstralh EJ, Kurland LT. Epidemiology and clinical features of idiopathic trigeminal neuralgia and glossopharyngeal neuralgia: similarities and differences, Rochester, Minnesota, 1945–1984. Neuroepidemiology.; 10(5–6):276–281

[3] Headache Classification Subcommittee of the International Headache Society. The International Classification of Headache Disorders, 3rd ed (beta version). Cephalalgia.; 33; 9: 629–808

[4] Shackleton T, Ram S, Black M, Ryder J, Clark GT, Enciso R. The efficacy of botulinum toxin for the treatment of trigeminal and postherpetic neuralgia: a systematic review with meta-analyses. Oral Surg Oral Med Oral Pathol Oral Radiol.; 122(1): 61–71

[5] Love S, Coakham HB. Trigeminal neuralgia: pathology and pathogenesis. Brain.; 124(Pt 12):2347–2360

[6] Barker FG, II, Jannetta PJ, Bissonette DJ, Larkins MV, Jho HD. The long-term outcome of microvascular decompression for trigeminal neuralgia. N Engl J Med.; 334(17):1077–1083

[7] Hilton DA, Love S, Gradidge T, Coakham HB. Pathological findings associated with trigeminal neuralgia caused by vascular compression. Neurosurgery.; 35(2):299–303, discussion 303

[8] Watson JC. From paroxysmal to chronic pain in trigeminal neuralgia: implications of central sensitization. Neurology.; 69(9):817–818

[9] Smith KJ, McDonald WI. Spontaneous and mechanically evoked activity due to central demyelinating lesion. Nature.; 286(5769):154–155

[10] Cruccu G, Gronseth G, Alksne J, et al. American Academy of Neurology Society, European Federation of Neurological Society. AAN-EFNS guidelines on trigeminal neuralgia management. Eur J Neurol.; 15(10):1013–1028

[11] Marino MJ, Terashima T, Steinauer JJ, Eddinger KA, Yaksh TL, Xu Q. Botulinum toxin B in the sensory afferent: transmitter release, spinal activation, and pain behavior. Pain.; 155(4): 674–684

[12] Cui M, Khanijou S, Rubino J, Aoki KR. Subcutaneous administration of botulinum toxin A reduces formalin-induced pain. Pain.; 107(1–2):125–133

[13] Türk U, Ilhan S, Alp R, Sur H. Botulinum toxin and intractable trigeminal neuralgia. Clin Neuropharmacol.; 28(4):161–162

[14] Piovesan EJ, Teive HG, Kowacs PA, Della Coletta MV, Werneck LC, Silberstein SD. An open study of botulinum-A toxin treatment of trigeminal neuralgia. Neurology.; 65(8): 1306–1308

[15] Boscá-Blasco ME, Burguera-Hernández JA, Roig-Morata S, Martínez-Torres I. [Painful tic convulsif and Botulinum toxin]. Rev Neurol.; 42(12):729–732

[16] Allam N, Brasil-Neto JP, Brown G, Tomaz C. Injections of botulinum toxin type a produce pain alleviation in intractable trigeminal neuralgia. Clin J Pain.; 21(2):182–184

[17] Morra ME, Elgebaly A, Elmaraezy A, et al. Therapeutic efficacy and safety of botulinum toxin A therapy in trigeminal neuralgia: a systematic review and meta-analysis of randomized controlled trials. J Headache Pain.; 17(1):63

[18] Safarpour Y, Jabbari B. Botulinum toxin treatment of pain syndromes -an evidence based review. Toxicon.; 147(1): 120–128

[19] Krafft RM. Trigeminal neuralgia. Am Fam Physician.; 77(9): 1291–1296

17
Botulinum Neurotoxin for Frey Syndrome

Rachel Kaye, Andrew Blitzer, and Brian E. Benson

Summary

Frey syndrome (FS) describes facial hyperhidrosis, erythema, or warmth encouraged by gustatory stimuli. It is due to aberrant regeneration of postganglionic parasympathetic fibers from the auriculotemporal nerve that reinnervate superficial facial eccrine sweat glands and cutaneous blood vessels. As such, vasodilation and localized sweating occur in response to mastication and salivary stimuli. Botulinum neurotoxin (BoNT) is the first line of therapy in patients with FS and boasts a good safety profile and excellent results. Although most patients require repeat injections, they also experience a greater time interval between injections compared to other syndromes that are treated with BoNT. The exact mechanism for this increased duration of symptomatic improvement is not understood. Further high-quality research is necessary to support the BoNT treatment strategy because, although it is the first-line therapy for FS, it is still currently being utilized in an "off-label" fashion.

Keywords: chemodenervation, botulinum toxin, Frey syndrome, gustatory sweating, auriculotemporal syndrome, hyperhidrosis

17.1 Introduction

Frey syndrome (FS), also known as gustatory sweating or auriculotemporal syndrome, is characterized by excessive facial sweating, erythema, and/or warmth that is stimulated by the thought, sight, or consumption of food. Although originally described in 1757 by Duphenix[1] and later in 1853 by Baillarger,[2] this syndrome is named after Lucja Frey, a Polish neurologist, who first described gustatory sweating following traumatic parotid injury in 1923 and coined the term "auriculotemporal syndrome."[3] This phenomenon typically occurs following surgery or trauma to the parotid gland, facial nerve, submandibular gland, or thoracic sympathetic chain. It can be associated with polyneuropathies which result in maladaptive parasympathetic cholinergic innervation of cutaneous sympathetic receptors.[4,5]

17.2 Etiology

Frey syndrome is thought to be due to aberrant regeneration of postganglionic parasympathetic fibers from the auriculotemporal nerve that reinnervate superficial facial eccrine sweat glands and cutaneous blood vessels.[6] Due to this faulty reinnervation, vasodilation and localized sweating occurs in response to gustatory stimuli. This phenomenon is usually due to trauma to these fibers or iatrogenic disruption following parotidectomy where these fibers are surgically separated and become aberrantly connected to the superficial vasculature and sweat glands. As nerve regeneration typically occurs 3 to 6 months following injury, this is the typical timeline for presentation to the physician with classic symptoms and conversion to a positive minor iodine starch test (MIST).[7]

A 2017 retrospective review of 100 patients with FS reported a history of parotidectomy in 96% with a minority of remaining cases due to trauma (2%) or mumps (1%).[7] Conversely, the rate of clinical prevalence of FS following parotidectomy ranges from 4 to 62%.[8] A 2011 study highlighted the subclinical nature of FS as the prevalence of a positive MIST was 62% in postparotidectomy patients, but only 23% reported symptoms.[9] Indeed, this corresponds well with the 1958 classic report that MIST can be positive in up to 100% of postparotidectomy patients, while only 15 to 30% report clinical symptoms.[10] This decline in incidence of positive MIST and FS over the past five decades may be due in part to improved understanding of the disorder and resultant prophylactic measures taken during parotidectomy, such as increased skin flap thickness, although this reasoning is unproven. Ultimately, FS remains the most common long-term self-perceived consequence of surgical intervention in patients undergoing parotidectomy for benign disease.[11]

17.3 Workup

A complete history and physical exam is necessary to elucidate the underlying pathology and initiate treatment planning. Symptoms such as flushing, sweating, burning, and pruritus are usually mild but can result in social anxiety, social isolation, and discomfort. Although the diagnosis is clinical, confirmatory testing is performed with the MIST. It is important to note that this test typically becomes positive 3 to 6 months after surgery. During the MIST, the suspected region is painted with a thin layer of povidone-iodine solution. After the solution dries, dried starch (a mixture of 10–20% amylose and 80–90% amylopectin) is applied to the painted area. An oral sialogogue (lemon juice, citrus candy, etc.) is then provided to the patient to stimulate the gustatory cortex. When hydrated with sweat, the iodine molecules form a linear polyiodide ion complex that binds to the inside of the amylose helical polymer. The amylose-iodine complex absorbs a different light wavelength than the polypeptide alone, and the complex becomes discolored (dark blue/brown). Typically, a punctate pattern of sweat will first appear in affected areas within the prepared field, followed by coalescence of the droplets into a solid blue region. Some areas will take longer to appear than others, and care should be taken to avoid dripping sweat from discoloring areas that are not exhibiting sweating (▶ Fig. 17.1).

An alternative to the MIST is medical infrared thermography. This technique allows for isolation not only of the area of hyperhidrosis but also that of local facial flushing.[12] However, at the time of this publication, thermography remains experimental and is not widely available for clinical use.

17.4 Treatment

Several treatment options exist, including antiperspirant therapy (such as aluminum

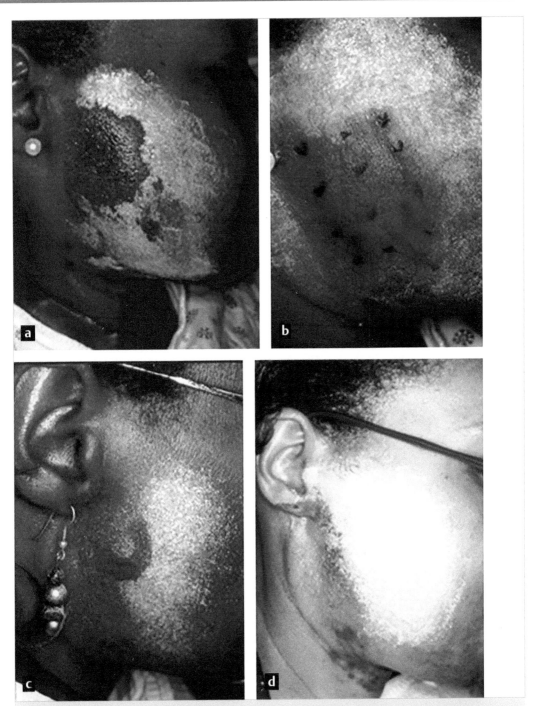

Fig. 17.1 Minor's starch-iodine test (MIST)-assisted treatment planning. (**a**) Initial MIST showing the darkened area of hyperhidrosis. (**b**) Planned injection points that encompass the entire effected area and occur 1 cm apart. (**c**) Repeat MIST 2 weeks following initial injection. The MIST is repeated for all subsequent injections to localize sites of recurrent/ persistent symptoms. (**d**) Repeat MIST 4 months following initial injection showing great and persistent response to botulinum neurotoxin chemodenervation.

chloride),[13] medical treatments, surgical techniques, and botulinum neurotoxin type A (BoNT-A). Topical antiperspirants, especially aluminum salts, form a plug in the acrosyringium (the superficial, intraepidermal portion of the sweat gland duct).[14] Local pruritus and skin irritation can occur with frequent application and antiperspirant therapy is considered suboptimal due to unclear long-term adverse effects and inability to achieve good dosage control during application. Similarly, topical medical therapy can include atropine or scopolamine hydrobromide ointment prior to meals.[10] However, the use of topical anticholinergic applications (i.e., glycopyrrolate solution) is limited by their systemic effects. Systemic oral anticholinergics (oxybutynin, glycopyrrolate, methantheline bromide, bornaprine hydrochloride) are usually only used when there is generalized hyperhidrosis or failure of local treatment.[14] Surgical therapies aim to create a separation barrier between the deep postganglionic parasympathetic nerve endings from the superficial cutaneous tissue. Such techniques include increased skin flap thickness, local rearrangement flaps, and the use of an interposition graft like acellular dermal matrix or autologous fat autotransplantation. However, overall the results have been suboptimal and BoNT injection is currently the first-line therapy for FS.

BoNT intracutaneous application for FS was first described in 1994[15] and more groups have reported similarly longstanding results using the same method in the past two decades.[16,17,18,19] As the toxin inhibits the presynaptic release of acetylcholine, it inhibits cholinergic nerve stimuli in a long-lasting but reversible manner. A 2015 review showed that clinical efficiency of BoNT for FS reached 98.5%. However, it is important to note that, to date, there has not yet been a study including a randomized control group, a feature that weakens the level of evidence.[20] Therefore, a 2015 Cochrane review ruled this intervention inconclusive due to lack of high-quality evidence.[21] Despite the lack of high-level evidence, BoNT has become widely accepted as both a safe and effective therapy for FS and other medications or surgical approaches are currently rarely used.[22]

For those who undergo BoNT therapy, most (70.5%) require repeat injections, with an average number for repeat injections being 5.8 and the average time interval between being 16.8 months.[7] Interestingly, the duration of effect for most studies is greater than 6 months[20] and has been shown to increase following repeat injections by some,[23] prompting others to posit that FS represents a dynamic process that can be modulated with BoNT therapy,[22] although this remains controversial.[20] Each patient should be counseled regarding the risks, benefits, and alternative therapies that exist for FS. If a patient desires to pursue BoNT injection, a detailed informed consent form must be completed which highlights that BoNT injection for FS is an "off-label" use of an approved medication.

17.5 Anatomy

The eccrine superficial facial sweat glands are normally stimulated by sympathetic innervation from the trigeminal nerve. Acetylcholine is the neurotransmitter responsible both for simulating parotid salivary production as well as eccrine gland activation.[24,25] As mentioned earlier, the aberrant and synkinetic reinnervation of severed parasympathetic fibers to the eccrine sweat glands and cutaneous vasculature occurs in FS. As both synaptic junctions are cholinergic, the aberrant regeneration results in skin flushing and hyperhidrosis upon salivary stimulation.

17.6 Technique

Although BoNT dosing varies depending on the size of the affected area, most authors report dosing amounts of 30 to 35 U per patient with slightly lower initiation dosing of 25 U.[7] Most studies advocate a concentration of 2.5 U/cm, an interinjection distance of 1 cm, and volume per injection point of 0.1 mL in the involved area.[8,20] The affected area is best confirmed by using a MIST prior to each treatment in order to tailor therapy (▶ Fig. 17.1). Although BoNT-A is the first-line therapy for FS, the B subtype (BoNT-B) has also shown clinical efficacy and can be used if patients become resistant to BoNT-A injection.[16]

Following MIST, a grid is marked on the skin using a makeup pencil with 1 cm markings throughout the areas of positivity on MIST (▶ Fig. 17.1b). BoNT-A is usually diluted to a concentration of 2.5 U/0.1 mL and is injected intradermally (not subcutaneously) via a 1-mL tuberculin syringe with either a 30- or 32-gauge needle. Injection points occur at each crosshatch or intersection of the grid pattern to allow for 1 cm of diffusion around each point. Following injection, the skin is cleaned and the patient is asked to return in 2 to 4 weeks to assess treatment response.

17.7 Follow-up

The MIST is repeated on follow up visits. Any persistent areas of gustatory sweating are reinjected using the same technique as outlined earlier. Maximal BoNT effect occurs at 10 to 14 days and as such, a given patient is scheduled for follow-up 2 to 4 weeks following their initial injection in order to monitor response. Our protocol is to perform a third treatment 4 to 8 months later if the patient is symptomatic with injection site location being again guided by repeat MIST.

17.8 Complications and Pitfalls

Few reported complications have been described over the past two decades,[20] and there have been no reports of major complications as a result of BoNT treatment of FS. Mild local facial weakness may occur due to diffusion of the toxin to masticator muscles such as the masseter or buccinators. However, given the superficial nature of injection and the posterior position of the bulk of the parotid gland, such events are unlikely to occur. Additional mild adverse effects include local injection site–related discomforts, such as ecchymosis, tenderness, and edema. Proper technique with avoidance of superficial vessels using a small gauge needle helps prevent these adverse effects.

17.9 Key Points/Pearls

- Frey syndrome (FS) is due to aberrant regeneration of postganglionic parasympathetic fibers from the auriculotemporal nerve that reinnervate superficial facial eccrine sweat glands and cutaneous blood vessels.
- In FS, vasodilation and localized sweating occur in response to mastication and salivary stimuli.
- Botulinum neurotoxin (BoNT) is currently the first-line therapy for FS and successfully treats most patients with a good safety profile.
- FS patients treated with BoNT experience longer-lasting effects than that which can be explained due to the pharmacokinetic duration of active BoNT and thus have a greater time

interval between injections than for other disorders treated with BoNT.

- Further research, specifically multicenter randomized controlled trials, is needed to generate high-level evidence to support this effective treatment strategy.

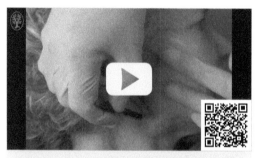

Video 17.1 Frey Syndrome. A Starch-Iodine test is first performed. This is done by painting the area of the face with iodine. Once dry, starch powder is dusted over the area. The patient is then given a sour lemon candy and as the sweat accumulated, it mixes the iodine and starch producing a dark area. Once delineated, a marking pen is then used to create a 1-cm grid. At each intersection of the grid, 2.5 U/0.1 cc of Botox is injected intradermally. The patient is brought back at two weeks and another Starch-Iodine test is done to see if there is any residual sweating. If so, additional toxin may be injected. [2:19]

References

[1] Duphenix M.. Observations sur les fistules du canal salivaire de Stenon: 1. Sur une playe compliquée á la joue ou le canal salivaire fut déchiré. Memoires de l'Académie Royale de Chirugie.; 3:431–439

[2] Baillarger JGF. Memoire sur l'obliteration du canal de Stenon. Gaz Med (Paris).; 23:194–197

[3] Frey L. Le syndrome du nerf auriculo-temporal. Rev Neurol (Paris).; 2:92–104

[4] Haxton HA. Gustatory sweating. Brain.; 71(1):16–25

[5] Spiro RH, Martin H. Gustatory sweating following parotid surgery and radical neck dissection. Ann Surg.; 165(1):118–127

[6] Gardner WJ, McCubbin JW. Auriculotemporal syndrome; gustatory sweating due to misdirection of regenerated nerve fibers. J Am Med Assoc.; 160(4):272–277

[7] Jansen S, Jerowski M, Ludwig L, Fischer-Krall E, Beutner D, Grosheva M. Botulinum toxin therapy in Frey's syndrome: a retrospective study of 440 treatments in 100 patients. Clin Otolaryngol.; 42(2):295–300

[8] Motz KM, Kim YJ. Auriculotemporal syndrome (Frey syndrome). Otolaryngol Clin North Am.; 49(2):501–509

[9] Neumann A, Rosenberger D, Vorsprach O, Dazert S. [The incidence of Frey syndrome following parotidectomy: results of a survey and follow-up]. HNO.; 59(2):173–178

[10] Laage-Hellman JE. Treatment of gustatory sweating and flushing. Acta Otolaryngol.; 49(2):132–143

[11] Baek CH, Chung MK, Jeong HS, et al. Questionnaire evaluation of sequelae over 5 years after parotidectomy for benign diseases. J Plast Reconstr Aesthet Surg.; 62(5):633–638

[12] Green RJ, Endersby S, Allen J, Adams J. Role of medical thermography in treatment of Frey's syndrome with botulinum toxin A. Br J Oral Maxillofac Surg.; 52(1):90–92

[13] Hüttenbrink KB. [Therapy of gustatory sweating following parotidectomy. Frey's syndrome]. Laryngol Rhinol Otol (Stuttg).; 65(3):135–137

[14] Hosp C, Naumann MK, Hamm H. Botulinum toxin treatment of autonomic disorders: focal hyperhidrosis and sialorrhea. Semin Neurol.; 36(1):20–28

[15] Drobik C, Laskawi R. Frey's syndrome: treatment with botulinum toxin. Acta Otolaryngol.; 115(3):459–461

[16] Cantarella G, Berlusconi A, Mele V, Cogiamanian F, Barbieri S. Treatment of Frey's syndrome with botulinum toxin type B. Otolaryngol Head Neck Surg.; 143(2):214–218

[17] Pomprasit M, Chintrakarn C. Treatment of Frey's syndrome with botulinum toxin. J Med Assoc Thai.; 90(11): 2397–2402

[18] Restivo DA, Lanza S, Patti F, et al. Improvement of diabetic autonomic gustatory sweating by botulinum toxin type A. Neurology.; 59(12):1971–1973

[19] Arad-Cohen A, Blitzer A. Botulinum toxin treatment for symptomatic Frey's syndrome. Otolaryngol Head Neck Surg.; 122(2):237–240

[20] Xie S, Wang K, Xu T, Guo XS, Shan XF, Cai ZG. Efficacy and safety of botulinum toxin type A for treatment of Frey's syndrome: evidence from 22 published articles. Cancer Med.; 4(11):1639–1650

[21] Li C, Wu F, Zhang Q, Gao Q, Shi Z, Li L. Interventions for the treatment of Frey's syndrome. Cochrane Database Syst Rev. (3):CD009959

[22] Steffen A, Rotter N, König IR, Wollenberg B. Botulinum toxin for Frey's syndrome: a closer look at different treatment responses. J Laryngol Otol.; 126(2):185–189

[23] de Bree R, Duyndam JE, Kuik DJ, Leemans CR. Repeated botulinum toxin type A injections to treat patients with Frey syndrome. Arch Otolaryngol Head Neck Surg.; 135(3): 287–290

[24] Valtorta F, Arslan G. The pharmacology of botulinum toxin. Pharmacol Res.; 27(1):33–44

[25] Sellin LC. The action of botulinum toxin at the neuromuscular junction. Med Biol.; 59(1):11–20

18
Botulinum Neurotoxin for Facial Hyperhidrosis

Diana N. Kirke, Daniel Novakovic, and Andrew Blitzer

Summary

Hyperhidrosis is characterized by excess perspiration and may be primary/idiopathic or secondary due to endocrine dysfunction, neoplasia, or chronic infection. There are several possible treatment modalities for this condition. Medical therapies include topical aluminum salts and anticholinergic medications; however, the use of these is limited by their side effects. Surgical treatments are effective yet are not without significant risk such as Horner syndrome and neuralgia. Finally, botulinum neurotoxin (BoNT) has been shown to be safe and a highly effective temporary treatment for idiopathic hyperhidrosis. Currently, onabotulinumtoxinA (Botox, Allergan plc, Irvine, CA) is the only formulation approved by the Food and Drug Administration for this condition. In this chapter, we will discuss the workup of patients presenting for treatment of hyperhidrosis, injection technique, as well as possible complications in order to provide a comprehensive review.

Keywords: botulinum neurotoxin, hyperhidrosis, neurologic disorders

18.1 Introduction

Hyperhidrosis is a common condition characterized by perspiration in excess of that required to regulate body temperature. It may be divided into primary and secondary forms. Primary (idiopathic or essential) hyperhidrosis is a focal disorder usually involving the palms, soles of feet, axillae, or face.[1,2] The onset of primary hyperhidrosis is usually during adolescence, and 30 to 50% of affected individuals report a positive family history, which suggests a genetic component. The genetic locus in primary palmar hyperhidrosis has been localized to chromosome 14.[3] Sweating episodes may be triggered by various factors including spicy foods, emotional stressors, and mental or physical activity, but do not occur during sleep. These episodes can cause significant social and occupational dysfunction, as well as psychological stress. Secondary hyperhidrosis is characterized by generalized perspiration and is usually related to excess adrenergic stimulation due to an underlying disease such as endocrine dysfunction, neoplasia, or chronic infection.[4] Autonomic dysfunction associated with neurologic disorders and medication side effects are less common causes. Gustatory hyperhidrosis (Frey syndrome) is a secondary focal variant most commonly seen after parotid gland surgery; it is discussed in Chapter 17.

Topical medical therapies for hyperhidrosis are available, but the results are often unsatisfactory. Topical aluminum salts in a concentration of 20 to 25% are an effective first-line treatment, but localized burning, stinging, and irritation may limit their use.[5] Iontophoresis is a second-line therapy that involves delivering ions through the skin using electrical current. Local irritation and the fact that it is time-consuming limit the use of this modality.

Systemic drugs are primarily indicated in the treatment of secondary hyperhidrosis. Anticholinergic medications, including glycopyrrolate, oxybutynin, propantheline bromide, and benztropine, have been used with some success. Unfortunately, due to the relatively large doses that are required, a significant side-effect profile exists. Common side effects, including dry mouth, blurred vision, tachycardia, and urinary retention, limit the clinical efficacy of oral anticholinergic medication.[6]

Surgical treatments can be effective but involve considerable risk. Endoscopic thoracic sympathectomy involves resection or ablation of the sympathetic ganglia. Reported response rates are high, with up to 86% of patients noting improvement in their quality of life.[7] The response appears to be lower in plantar hyperhidrosis. The usefulness of surgery is limited by a high incidence of compensatory hyperhidrosis usually on the torso and lower limbs in up to 86% of patients.[6] In addition, there is the risk of other more serious complications including Horner syndrome and neuralgia.[5] Other surgical therapies exist, such as removal of axillary glandular tissue, but are not appropriate in the craniofacial region.

Botulinum neurotoxin (BoNT) irreversibly blocks presynaptic acetylcholine release at the neuromuscular junction, thus exerting its muscular paralysis effects. Because acetylcholine is also the primary neurotransmitter responsible for transmission at the cholinergic neurosecretory junction, BoNT has also been shown to be a safe and highly effective method of abolishing focal sweating in idiopathic hyperhidrosis. BoNT exerts its effects in a similar way by cleaving presynaptic SNARE proteins at two different sites. All of the A toxins cleave SNAP-25, and the B toxin cleaves VAMP. In comparison to effects on muscle, BoNT has a longer duration of action in inhibiting glandular secretion, a phenomenon that is poorly understood, but is likely due to glandular atrophy.[8] OnabotulinumtoxinA (Botox, Allergan plc, Irvine, CA) was initially described for palmar hyperhidrosis but is also used commonly for axillary hyperhidrosis and is the only BoNT approved by the Food and Drug Administration (FDA) for the treatment of hyperhidrosis.[9,10,11,12,13] However, incobotulinumtoxinA (Xeomin, Merz North America Inc, Greensborough, NC), abobotulinumtoxinA (Dysport, Galderma Laboratories L.P., Fort Worth, TX), and other type A toxins currently in trials will likely show similar activity.

Böger et al[14] reported on the use of BoNT for idiopathic craniofacial hyperhidrosis. In this study, the diagnosis was confirmed with Minor's starch-iodine test. One half of the forehead (and the associated temple) received injections of intracutaneous onabotulinumtoxinA (Medicis Pharmaceutical, Scottsdale, AZ) in 0.1-ng aliquots using the contralateral side as a control. Some 25 to 40 injections were administered depending on the size of the region. The contralateral side was then treated 4 weeks later. Eleven of 12 patients reported complete resolution of their symptoms. All patients had some degree of forehead weakness, with two patients reporting temporary brow asymmetry (lasting up to 16 weeks). Only one patient had relapsed at 9 months.[15]

Both onabotulinumtoxinA (BoNT-A) and onabotulinumtoxinB (BoNT-B) are effective in the treatment of hyperhidrosis. There are some pharmacologic differences between the two subtypes. There is evidence that BoNT-B has a faster onset of action and that the autonomic nervous system is relatively more sensitive to BoNT-B compared with BoNT-A.[13] However, Rystedt et al[16] investigated the effects of BoNT-A and BoNT-B on sudomotor cholinergic function and found that BoNT-A was the most potent, achieving a mean anhidrotic area per unit of $0.69\,cm^2$ at the optimal concentration of 25 units (U)/mL. Furthermore, patients tend to report more discomfort with BoNT-B, probably due to its acidity.[16,17] Glogau suggested that the diffusion characteristics of BoNT-B were better than those of BoNT-A for axillary and palmar hyperhidrosis in that it diffuses more evenly.[18]

Despite the possible greater autonomic affinity of BoNT-B, we do not routinely employ it for facial hyperhidrosis. Its duration of action tends to be shorter than that of BoNT-A, and its greater diffusion may lead to more locoregional side effects in the head and neck, including dry mouth, mydriasis, dry eyes, and facial muscular weakness. Several studies have also suggested that BoNT-B produces more systemic side effects when compared with BoNT-A.[17]

18.2 Workup

A comprehensive history is essential to distinguish primary from secondary hyperhidrosis. The history should include the location of sweating, age at onset, causative factors, and family history, as well as a review of systems aimed at identifying associated symptoms that may indicate a possible secondary etiology. Generalized hyperhidrosis should prompt referral for endocrine workup, which may include thyroid function tests and catecholamine levels. The diagnosis of focal idiopathic hyperhidrosis can be confirmed by a starch-iodine test, which, although not strictly necessary, allows correct mapping of the affected areas and identification of problem areas requiring further injections in the event of treatment failure.

18.3 Anatomy

Eccrine glands are responsible for the production of sweat: a clear, odorless, hypotonic fluid. The gland itself is a long-branched structure with a coiled secretory region and a straight ductal region.[1,2] Eccrine glands are found in highest concentration on the soles of the hands and feet, closely followed by the forehead, axillae, and cheeks. They are innervated by cholinergic fibers from the sympathetic nervous system and assist with regulation of body temperature.

18.4 Technique

The patient is seated comfortably in a reclining chair. The selection of treatment areas is based on patient history and physical examination identifying the most active regions. A starch-iodine test may optionally be performed to improve accuracy (see Chapter 17). In the active areas of hyperhidrosis, a $1 \times 1\,cm$ grid is drawn using marker pencil or eyeliner (▶ Fig. 18.1). Local anesthesia is not routinely used. Injections are administered using a 1-mL tuberculin syringe attached to a 32-gauge needle.

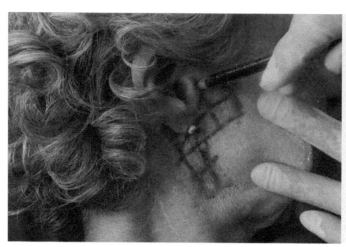

Fig. 18.1 Marking a 1 × 1 cm injection grid of the hypersecretory region.

OnabotulinumtoxinA is used in a dilution of 2.5 U per 0.1 mL, as this concentration has been shown to have the most enhanced anticholinergic effect.[16] Aliquots of 0.1 mL are delivered to the dermal–subcutaneous junction to each point on the grid where the lines intersect.[19] Special attention must be paid to creating the characteristic intradermal "bleb" with each injection, unlike the subcutaneous "wheal" commonly created during intramuscular facial injections. Excessive pressure is to be avoided to minimize diffusion into underlying musculature. The forehead region is typically treated first, as it has the highest concentration of eccrine glands and is the most common area of excess sweat production. The average dose for this region is approximately 40 U. For nasal and upper lip hyperhidrosis, the average dose is 10 U.[19]

18.5 Follow-up

Patients are reviewed at 3 weeks to monitor progress and adverse effects. Further "touch-up" injections can be administered at this point using the same technique with the aid of a starch-iodine test. After a satisfactory response, follow-up is on an as-required basis.

18.6 Complications and Pitfalls

Diffusion to the underlying musculature causing associated paralysis may occur as a side effect of treatment. In the forehead region, this phenomenon is almost universal, but is usually of little clinical significance.[14] Care must be taken to avoid asymmetry of the brow or active forehead movement. In addition, injection too close to the lateral brow may cause ptosis. Thus, the forehead region lateral to the pupil and within 2 cm of the eyebrow should be avoided. The middle and lower face should be approached with increased caution, due to the possibility of adversely affecting cosmesis and function associated with underlying facial musculature. In particular, when treating the nose, injections should be kept as medial as possible in order to avoid diffusion to the nasal musculature. Furthermore, patients should be warned that treating the upper lip may result in dropped lip, decreased pursing of the lips, and thus decreased oral competence.[19] Careful intradermal injection results in improved efficacy and decreased unwanted side effects. A thorough history and physical examination are important to identify symptoms and signs of secondary hyperhidrosis.

18.7 Conclusion

Botulinum neurotoxin is a safe, effective, durable, and reliable treatment with minimal unwanted side effects when used for facial hyperhidrosis in symptomatic patients who have failed more conservative medical treatment and do not wish to undergo surgery.

18.8 Key Points/Pearls

- Botulinum neurotoxin (BoNT) has been shown to be safe and a highly effective temporary treatment for idiopathic hyperhidrosis.
- Currently onabotulinumtoxinA (Botox, Allergan plc, Irvine, CA) is the only formulation approved by the FDA for this condition.
- Both onabotulinumtoxinA (BoNT-A) and onabotulinumtoxinB (BoNT-B) are effective; however, we generally do not use BoNT-B as there is suggestion that it may produce more side effects than BoNT-A.
- The average dose for the forehead region is 40 U, while the average dose for nasal and upper lip hyperhidrosis is 10 U.

References

[1] Kreyden OP, Scheidegger EP. Anatomy of the sweat glands, pharmacology of botulinum toxin, and distinctive syndromes associated with hyperhidrosis. Clin Dermatol.; 22(1):40–44

[2] Trindade de Almeida AR, Hexsel DM. Hyperhidrosis and Botulinum Toxin. Sao Paulo: A.R.T. Almeida; 2004

[3] Higashimoto I, Yoshiura K, Hirakawa N, et al. Primary palmar hyperhidrosis locus maps to 14q11.2-q13. Am J Med Genet A.; 140(6):567–572

[4] Böni R. Generalized hyperhidrosis and its systemic treatment. Curr Probl Dermatol.; 30:44–47

[5] Haider A, Solish N. Focal hyperhidrosis: diagnosis and management. CMAJ.; 172(1):69–75

[6] Connolly M, de Berker D. Management of primary hyperhidrosis: a summary of the different treatment modalities. Am J Clin Dermatol.; 4(10):681–697

[7] de Campos JR, Kauffman P, Werebe E de C, et al. Quality of life, before and after thoracic sympathectomy: report on 378 operated patients. Ann Thorac Surg.; 76(3):886–891

[8] Dressler D, Adib Saberi F, Benecke R. Botulinum toxin type B for treatment of axillar hyperhidrosis. J Neurol.; 249(12): 1729–1732

[9] Shelley WB, Talanin NY, Shelley ED. Botulinum toxin therapy for palmar hyperhidrosis. J Am Acad Dermatol.; 38(2, Pt 1): 227–229

[10] Naumann M, Flachenecker P, Bröcker E-B, Toyka KV, Reiners K. Botulinum toxin for palmar hyperhidrosis. Lancet.; 349 (9047):252

[11] Schnider P, Binder M, Auff E, Kittler H, Berger T, Wolff K. Double-blind trial of botulinum A toxin for the treatment of focal hyperhidrosis of the palms. Br J Dermatol.; 136(4):548–552

[12] Bushara KO, Park DM. Botulinum toxin and sweating. J Neurol Neurosurg Psychiatry.; 57(11):1437–1438

[13] Bushara KO, Park DM, Jones JC, Schutta HS. Botulinum toxin—a possible new treatment for axillary hyperhidrosis. Clin Exp Dermatol.; 21(4):276–278

[14] Böger A, Herath H, Rompel R, Ferbert A. Botulinum toxin for treatment of craniofacial hyperhidrosis. J Neurol.; 247(11): 857–861

[15] Nicholas R, Quddus A, Baker DM. Treatment of primary craniofacial hyperhidrosis: a systematic review. Am J Clin Dermatol.; 16(5):361–370

[16] Rystedt A, Swartling C, Naver H. Anhidrotic effect of intradermal injections of botulinum toxin: a comparison of different products and concentrations. Acta Derm Venereol.; 88(3): 229–233

[17] Baumann LS, Halem ML. Botulinum toxin-B and the management of hyperhidrosis. Clin Dermatol.; 22(1):60–65

[18] Glogau RG. Review of the use of botulinum toxin for hyperhidrosis and cosmetic purposes. Clin J Pain.; 18(6) Suppl: S191–S197

[19] Glaser DA, Galperin TA. Botulinum toxin for hyperhidrosis of areas other than the axillae and palms/soles. Dermatol Clin.; 32(4):517–525

19 Botulinum Neurotoxin for Sialorrhea

Brianna K. Crawley, Scott M. Rickert, Senja Tomovic, and Andrew Blitzer

Summary

Sialorrhea can be a debilitating sequela of some neurologic disorders. Botulinum neurotoxin (BoNT) infiltration into the major salivary glands is a good noninvasive option to help decrease the amount of saliva production. Here, we describe the anatomy, interventions, and techniques for using BoNT for sialorrhea.

Keywords: sialorrhea, parotid, submandibular, ultrasound guidance, Parkinson disease, amyotrophic lateral sclerosis, parotitis

19.1 Introduction

Sialorrhea is defined as salivation beyond the lip margin. Sialorrhea is considered normal in infants, and it typically stops in the second year of life. Sialorrhea is considered pathologic when it presents in patients who are 4 years of age or older. Sialorrhea is a common disorder found in adult patients with neurologic deficits (stroke, amyotrophic lateral sclerosis [ALS], Parkinson disease [PD]) and in children and adults who are neurologically impaired (cerebral palsy, mental retardation, etc.). It is predominantly due to poor oral/facial muscular control in combination with hypersecretion, poor posture, and poor occlusion.

In a normal adult, approximately 1.5 L of saliva is produced daily. The six major salivary glands—the bilateral parotid, submandibular, and sublingual glands—produce 90% of the total saliva. Hundreds of minor salivary glands throughout the oral cavity and oropharynx produce the rest. At baseline, approximately 70% of the total production comes from the submandibular and sublingual glands. When fully stimulated, the salivary production can increase five times, with the parotid gland production increasing dramatically.[1] Saliva is important for oral function and health by lubricating food boluses, providing amylase for initial food breakdown, and preventing local infection through its bacteriostatic and bacteriocidal properties.

The neurologic pathways for salivation arise from the parasympathetic nervous system, which originates its signals in the pons and medulla. The preganglionic fibers synapse in the otic and submandibular ganglions and then travel postganglionically to the parotid gland (via the otic ganglion) and the submandibular and sublingual (via the submandibular ganglion). Sympathetic muscular contraction enhances the expression of saliva when stimulated.

The complications associated with sialorrhea include dehydration, foul odor, and poor oral/perioral hygiene, which can lead to frequent local infections. These complications lead to many psychosocial issues such as isolation, poor social standing, and further dependency of care, and provide barriers to normal socialization (unable to share toys due to excess salivation). As these patients typically have other pressing medical issues as well, sialorrhea is frequently overlooked as a potentially treatable problem. A team approach to sialorrhea,[2] including providers from primary care, dentistry, neurology, otolaryngology, and occupational therapy, has been shown to result in improved outcomes.

There are several different etiologies of sialorrhea, often acting in combination: neuromuscular dysfunction, hypersecretion, sensory dysfunction, and motor dysfunction. PD is the most common etiology in adults. Pseudobulbar palsy, bulbar palsy, facial nerve paralysis, and stroke are less common causes. In children, cerebral palsy and mental retardation are the most common etiologies.

Hypersecretion is typically caused by teething, dental caries, or oral infections. Medications, reflux, and toxins are other possible causes of hypersecretion. Poor swallowing function is seen frequently in patients with PD. Anatomic abnormalities such as macroglossia and malocclusion, surgical changes, and neurologic changes such as facial paralysis all can adversely affect oral competence and management of increased secretions.

19.2 Workup

Evaluation of sialorrhea should include a thorough history and physical examination to characterize the severity and frequency as well as measure the degree of detriment to the patient's quality of life. Noting the characteristics of the drooling—its consistency and flow patterns throughout the daytime on a typical day—is important to help formulate an effective treatment plan.

A comprehensive head and neck examination, with specific emphasis on the neurologic component, is crucial in devising a successful treatment plan. Head position, tongue size, tonsil size, adenoid size, perioral skin condition, dental health, mandibular position, malocclusion, nasal obstruction, and the presence of mouth breathing are important anatomic factors. Neurologic signs such as tongue thrusting, hyposensitive and hypersensitive gag reflex, swallowing inefficiencies, laryngeal hyposensitivity and hypersensitivity, and tongue mobility are very important to note. Flexible nasopharyngeal laryngoscopy is an important component of the examination to fully assess the upper airway for anatomic or neurologic abnormalities.

Sialorrhea can be measured by subjective scales and objective measures (▶ Table 19.1).

19.3 Anatomy

Sialorrhea predominantly comes from the major salivary glands: the bilateral parotid glands and the bilateral submandibular glands (▶ Fig. 19.1). The submandibular glands lie superior to the digastric muscles in the anterior neck. There is a superficial and deep lobe associated with each gland, which is separated by the mylohyoid muscle. Typically, the deep lobe contains the majority of the gland. Secretions emanate from the gland and follow Wharton's duct on the gland's superior surface, crossing the lingual nerve and traveling anteriorly to drain just lateral to the lingual frenulum in the floor of the mouth.

Table 19.1 Subjective scales and objective measures of sialorrhea

Subjective scales of sialorrhea	
1.	Drooling quotient (DQ): 40 observations in 10 hours DQ = percent of observations with drooling present
2.	Teacher drooling scale: 1 = no drooling 3 = occasional drooling 5 = constant wet saliva leaking on clothing/furniture
3.	Thomas-Stonell/Greenberg Assessment of Drooling[3]: Severity: 1 = dry 2 = mild (wet lips) 3 = moderate (wet lips/chin) 4 = severe (damp clothing) 5 = profuse (clothing, hands, furniture are wet) Frequency: 1 = never drools 2 = occasionally drools 3 = frequently drools 4 = constant drools
4.	Wilkie and Brody assessment of drooling[4]: Excellent: normal salivary control Good: slight loss of saliva ± dried lips Fair: significant residual saliva loss or perioral thickened froth Poor: failure to control/too dry
Objective measures of sialorrhea	
1.	Radioisotope scanning[5]: collection at chin for designated time period
2.	Salivary flow rate (mL/min): use of dental rolls at orifice, and measurement of weight difference after designated time period

The parotid glands lie between the zygomatic arch and the angle of the mandible just anterior-inferior to the external ear. It is shaped as a pyramid directed inferiorly. Landmarks near the parotid include the styloid process medially, the posterior belly of the digastrics medially and inferiorly, the mandible anteriorly, and the sternocleidomastoid posteriorly. Three major structures run through the parotid gland: the facial nerve and its associated branches, which separate the superior lobe from the deep lobe of the parotid; the maxillary and superficial temporal artery branches of the external carotid artery; and the retromandibular vein.

Salivary flow from minor ductal structures coalesces in Stensen's duct and drains medially and anteriorly to the oral mucosal orifice just adjacent to the second upper molar bilaterally.

19.4 Technique

A team approach to the treatment of sialorrhea is typically the most successful.[1] Occupational therapists and speech pathologists work to improve the swallowing mechanics and help provide posture support through exercises or devices such as the head-back wheelchair. The dentist treats any malocclusion issues as well as oral decay. Orthodontic appliances or customized palate inserts can aid in better oral competence. The primary care and social work team works to improve basic quality-of-life issues that impact the patient. The otolaryngology team works to correct any anatomic abnormalities such as adenotonsillar hypertrophy, nasal obstruction, and macroglossia that may contribute to sialorrhea. Neurologists help identify any neuropathologies associated with sialorrhea to plan appropriate oral medications that would aid in the treatment plan.

When all of the team members have met to discuss the patient's various problems, an overall plan of treatment is devised with the patient's input. Treatment options range from conservative (observation, postural changes, biofeedback treatment) to more aggressive measures of medication, radiation, and surgical therapy.

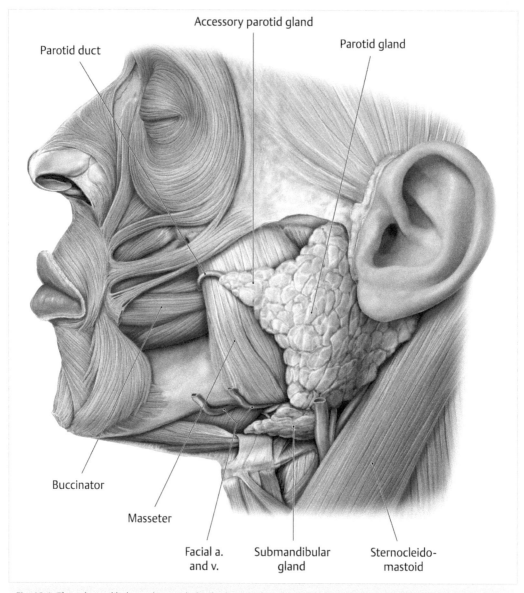

Accessory parotid gland

Parotid gland

Parotid duct

Buccinator

Masseter

Facial a. and v.

Submandibular gland

Sternocleido-mastoid

Fig. 19.1 The submandibular and parotid glands. (From Schuenke M, Schulte E, Schumacher U. THIEME Atlas of Anatomy: Head, Neck, and Neuroanatomy. Illustrations by Voll M and Wesker K. 2nd Ed. New York: Thieme Medical Publishers; 2016.)

Anticholinergic medications are effective in reducing drooling, but can be limited by side effects. BoNT-A injections into the parotid and submandibular glands are safe and effective,[6] but repeat injections are necessary as the effect is temporary. Surgical intervention, including salivary gland excision, salivary duct ligation, and duct rerouting, provides the most effective, permanent treatment of significant sialorrhea to improve the patient's quality of life.[7] Typically, the treatment begins with the least invasive option, and progresses, if necessary, to more aggressive options.

19.4.1 Noninvasive Techniques

Observation is an option for patients with minimal issues or with unstable neurologic function.[1] Children under the age of 4 are also typically observed if the sialorrhea is not significant. Feeding programs and exercises geared toward better oromotor control can be initiated for those able to follow a program.

Biofeedback has been shown to be successful in patients with mild neurologic deficits related to sialorrhea and in patients over 8 years of age.[8] The drawback is that these patients typically become habituated to the feedback, with less efficacy over time if the device feedback is not altered.[9] Further positive and negative reinforcement can help as an adjunct method to provide sialorrhea control. These measures usually result in mild improvement.[10]

Plates can be designed to aid in better lip closure[11,12] for those with poor closure. Beads can be placed on the upper plate and can also be used to stimulate tongue movement and redirect saliva toward the pharynx with moderate success.[13,14]

Acupuncture of the tongue has shown a limited subjective improvement in a small study.[15] Although further study is warranted, this modality is a minimally invasive technique for those unable to tolerate more invasive methods.

If none of these noninvasive methods ameliorate the sialorrhea, then it may be necessary to proceed to more invasive techniques such as oral medications, BoNT, radiation treatment, and surgical intervention.

19.4.2 Anticholinergic Medication

Anticholinergic medications work by blocking the parasympathetic innervation of the salivary flow. Both glycopyrrolate and scopolamine have been shown to be effective. As always, anticholinergics are contraindicated in patients with glaucoma, obstructive uropathy, gastrointestinal motility disorders, or myasthenia gravis, and are frequently poorly tolerated in elderly patients. Unfortunately, both glycopyrrolate and scopolamine also have side-effect profiles that are so severe that over 30% of patients are unable to tolerate these medications. For example, 23% of patients taking glycopyrrolate have significant behavioral changes,[16] and a significant number of patients taking scopolamine or glycopyrrolate note urinary retention and blurred vision.[16,17]

19.4.3 Botulinum Neurotoxin Injection Technique

Because of the relatively high side-effect profile for anticholinergic medications, BoNT is the primary modality in the nonsurgical treatment of sialorrhea. It not only blocks acetylcholine release at the neuromuscular synaptic end plate, but also blocks cholinergic parasympathetic secretomotor fibers of the salivary glands. There have been several series and randomized controlled clinical trials assessing the ability of BoNT to ameliorate sialorrhea in patients with various neurological disorders. The vast majority have shown significant benefit by subjective patient-reported outcome improvement and objective reduction of saliva production. A systematic review by Dashtipour et al synthesizes the most current data, evaluating six randomized controlled trials of BoNT for sialorrhea in patients with PD and ALS. The sample size ranged from 9 to 54 patients, injections ranged from 1,000 to 4,000 units (U) of BoNT-B or 250 U of BoNT-A, injections were performed into the parotid and submandibular glands, and follow-up varied from 4 to 16 weeks. The results showed statistically significant improvement in subjective and objective measures of sialorrhea and minimal side effects. Though there are limitations in power and variability in dosage, technique, and follow-up, this clearly shows strong evidence to support the efficacy and safety in BoNT for sialorrhea.[18] Another recent review of long-term data and literature found similar statistically significant positive results in the subjective and objective reduction of sialorrhea. It also highlighted that older patients had a benefit for a longer time and patients with PD had a favorable safety:efficacy ratio as compared to ALS patients.[19] There has also been increasing use of BoNT in salivary gland fistulas, in order to help improve outcomes, decrease healing time, and decrease need for more invasive interventions.[20,21]

The potential side-effect profile includes xerostomia, change in saliva thickness, mild transient dysphagia, mild weakness of chewing, neck pain, and diarrhea. These symptoms can be dose dependent, inaccurate needle placement, or diffusion into local muscles. The concern of decreased saliva causing changes in oral health seems to be relatively unfounded. The risk of increased dental caries has not been reported and furthermore a study showed no significant changes in salivary composition or carcinogenic bacterial counts pre- and 1-month post-BoNT-A injection.[22]

Typical doses reported in the literature range from 5 to 50 U of BoNT-A (or rough equivalent) per gland. In our practice, we have found that moderate doses injected with ultrasound guidance, and follow-up injections as necessary, have provided satisfactory results. Although BoNT can be injected solely into the parotid gland, it has been noted to be more successful at controlling sialorrhea when injected into both the submandibular and parotid glands. Injections may be performed using "blind" palpation of the gland, EMG guidance, or ultrasound guidance. Some authors feel that the use of ultrasound in injecting botulinum reduces the risks of complications.[23] When injecting with EMG guidance, the EMG is used to avoid intramuscular injection. In the case of the submandibular gland, audible action potentials heard after the gland has been entered likely reflect activity of the mylohyoid muscle, and indicate that the needle tip has passed beyond the substance of the gland. When injecting with ultrasound guidance, the needle can be visualized, the motion of the adjacent tissue can be appreciated, and a small test "wheal" will be clearly visible at the site of the needle tip (▶ Fig. 19.2, ▶ Fig. 19.3).

For the aforementioned reasons, the authors recommend ultrasound-guided injection of the submandibular glands, which can be more difficult to palpate. The location of the gland adjacent to multiple muscles of deglutition increases the risk of inadvertent injection or diffusion of the BoNT, thereby causing dysphagia in a population often already at risk for dysphagia, prior to chemodenervation of the submandibular glands.

The overall preponderance of the literature supports the use of BoNT injection as a safe and effective treatment for sialorrhea. However, it is important to note that the ideal dose, the best type of BoNT, and the most effective injection method have not yet been identified. Repeated injections are necessary for long-term control, typically on the order of every 4 months (for BoNT-A).

Techniques of Botulinum Neurotoxin Injection for Sialorrhea

Once the anatomy had been identified, the patient is superficially anesthetized with either topical lidocaine cream or injectable 1% lidocaine with epinephrine (1:100,000). The gland is palpated in one hand and the needle is directed into the substance of the gland. Careful intraoral counterpressure may be helpful, if the gland is difficult to palpate. BoNT is slowly injected throughout the substance of the gland until the desired amount of toxin is reached. If the gland is not easily palpated, ultrasonic guidance is very useful to help guide the injection. As long as the injection is within the substance of the gland, the risk of diffusion of toxin to local musculature is low. A slow injection reduces the diffusion pressures and helps minimize this risk.

Ultrasound-guided injection gives added reassurance of correct injection placement and visual confirmation of adequate distribution. The overlying skin is

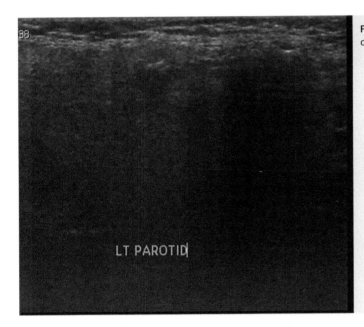

Fig. 19.2 Ultrasound-guided injection of the parotid gland.

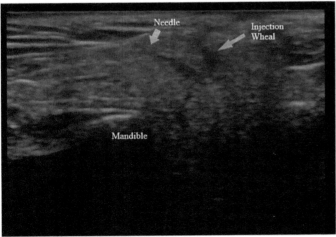

Fig. 19.3 Ultrasound-guided injection of the left parotid gland. Arrows depicting needle and infiltration wheal.

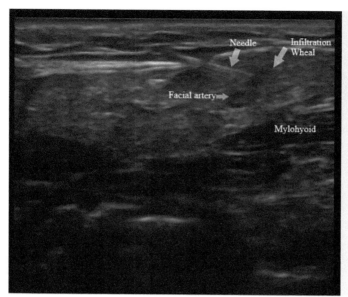

Fig. 19.4 Ultrasound-guided injection of the right submandibular gland. Arrows depicting needle and infiltration wheal and key structure that are visualized and avoided: the mylohyoid and facial artery.

cleaned with ethanol. The glands are first visualized and inspected with the covered ultrasound probe. A 25-gauge needle is then guided into the gland under ultrasound visualization. When it is confirmed to be in adequate position in the parenchyma of the gland, and not in musculature or vessels, the BoNT is slowly infiltrated and a wheal is visualized (▶ Fig. 19.3, ▶ Fig. 19.4).

The needle can then be advanced or repositioned with ultrasound guidance. We typically start with 17.5 to 25 U of BoNT-A per submandibular gland and 25 to 50 U per parotid gland. The dosing can be adjusted as needed for patient-reported symptoms. In the author's experience, a large bulk of parotid tissue exists in the tail region, especially as the glands atrophy, and ultrasound helps visualize this region more precisely.

19.4.4 Radiation Therapy

Aside from BoNT injections, radiation treatment to the salivary glands is another option for those patients unable to tolerate medical treatment or more aggressive surgical treatment.[24] The dose can be titrated to the desired effect, as radiation treatment causes xerostomia. Because potential malignancies typically do not occur for 15 to 20 years after the radiation therapy, this therapy is reserved for patients who are debilitated and elderly.[24]

19.4.5 Surgical Treatment

There are several potential surgical treatments for sialorrhea including salivary duct rerouting, salivary duct ligation, salivary gland excision, and surgery to denervate the salivary glands. Typically, surgical intervention involves some combination of the aforementioned methods to provide a more complete and permanent solution for sialorrhea.

Submandibular or parotid duct relocation is helpful to redirect the salivary flow posteriorly to limit sialorrhea. This method can cause potential dental caries and increased risk of aspiration, but it avoids external incisions.

Tympanic neurectomy can be performed to denervate the salivary glands at the tympanic plexus in the middle ear. This is a relatively straightforward procedure and can be done with the patient under mild sedation. Due to proximity to the chorda tympani, loss of taste is a rare side effect. This intervention is usually temporary, as the nerve fibers regenerate their pathways in 12 to 18 months.[25]

Excision of the submandibular glands is the most effective method to control sialorrhea and is a mainstay of surgical treatment. Typically, this procedure is performed via an external incision. Facial nerve injury, specifically the marginal mandibular nerve, is always a risk in submandibular gland excision, but the recent advent of facial nerve monitoring and the presence of good anatomic landmarks limit the risks. The most definitive surgical procedure combines the submandibular gland excision and parotid duct relocation or parotid duct ligation to limit the parotid salivary flow. It is highly successful in controlling sialorrhea, and it entails only a low incidence of facial weakness, with an improvement in the patient's quality of life.[7] Those patients who have failed other treatment options have found good success with this most aggressive of treatments for sialorrhea.

19.5 Emerging Uses of Botulinum Neurotoxin in the Salivary Glands

The use of BoNT has expanded and recently it has been explored in the context of parotitis. These uses have been described only in case reports, but it is worth mentioning as a new horizon for the treatment of some of these recalcitrant and progressive diseases.

A few studies examined the use of BoNT in Sjögren syndrome–related recurrent parotitis.[26,27] The underlying mechanism of recurrent parotitis in Sjögren syndrome involves sialectasis due to lymphocyte infiltration of the gland and ductal system, causing salivary stasis which can lead to inflammation and infection. The accumulation of saliva can then result in inflammation and infection. By reducing the amount of saliva accumulation with BoNT, physicians have been able to decrease the symptoms of parotitis and number of antibiotic treatments needed.[26,27] In addition, there is one report of BoNT use for symptomatic salivary gland ductal stenosis that failed ductal dilation and in lieu of sialadenectomy.[28] In all these cases, postobstructive sialadenitis was treated with BoNT as a less invasive reduced risk profile alternative to sialadenectomy when other interventions fail.

19.6 Conclusion

Sialorrhea is a common problem found in both adult and pediatric populations with neurologic disorders. It is important to understand the patient's specific quality-of-life issues to better devise a treatment strategy in a team approach. Noninvasive methods, such as observation, postural changes, and biofeedback, can aid mild cases. However, more severe cases typically require medical, radiation, or surgical treatment. BoNT injection into the salivary glands is an effective and safe short-term solution that requires repeated injections on a 3- to 4-month basis. Radiation treatment is reserved for poor surgical and medical candidates. Surgical interventions such as salivary duct rerouting, salivary duct ligation, tympanic neurectomy, and salivary gland excision are reserved for severe cases in which more conservative treatments have failed or prolonged neurologic dysfunction is expected.

19.7 Key Points/Pearls

- Sialorrhea is caused by a combination of neuromuscular dysfunction, hypersecretion, sensory dysfunction, and motor dysfunction.
- A treatment team involving primary care providers, dentists, neurologists, otolaryngologists, and occupational therapists improves treatment outcomes.
- Noninvasive techniques including postural changes, biofeedback, and dental appliances are treatment options for mild sialorrhea. The utility of oral anticholinergic medications is limited by adverse side effects.
- Botulinum toxin is the primary nonsurgical treatment of sialorrhea, achieving temporary subjective and objective reduction of sialorrhea. Results are improved by ultrasound guidance and repeat injections.
- Surgical intervention including salivary gland excision and salivary duct ligation or rerouting is effective in providing a permanent treatment for sialorrhea.

References

[1] Stuchell RN, Mandel ID. Salivary gland dysfunction and swallowing disorders. Otolaryngol Clin North Am.; 21(4): 649–661

[2] Crysdale WS. Drooling. Experience with team assessment and management. Clin Pediatr (Phila).; 31(2):77–80

[3] Thomas-Stonell N, Greenberg J. Three treatment approaches and clinical factors in the reduction of drooling. Dysphagia.; 3 (2):73–78

[4] Wilkie TF. The problem of drooling in cerebral palsy: a surgical approach. Can J Surg.; 10(1):60–67

[5] Sochaniwskyj AE. Drool quantification: noninvasive technique. Arch Phys Med Rehabil.; 63(12):605–607

[6] Hockstein NG, Samadi DS, Gendron K, Handler SD. Sialorrhea: a management challenge. Am Fam Physician.; 69(11): 2628–2634

[7] Shott SR, Myer CM, III, Cotton RT. Surgical management of sialorrhea. Otolaryngol Head Neck Surg.; 101(1):47–50

[8] Domaracki LS, Sisson LA. Decreasing drooling with oral motor stimulation in children with multiple disabilities. Am J Occup Ther.; 44(8):680–684

[9] Lancioni GE, Brouwer JA, Coninx F. Automatic cueing to reduce drooling: a long-term follow-up with two mentally handicapped persons. J Behav Ther Exp Psychiatry.; 25(2): 149–152

[10] Thorbecke PJ, Jackson HJ. Reducing chronic drooling in a retarded female using a multi-treatment package. J Behav Ther Exp Psychiatry.; 13(1):89–93

[11] Asher RS, Winquist H. Appliance therapy for chronic drooling in a patient with mental retardation. Spec Care Dentist.; 14 (1):30–32

[12] Hoyer H, Limbrock GJ. Orofacial regulation therapy in children with Down syndrome, using the methods and appliances of Castillo-Morales. ASDC J Dent Child.; 57(6):442–444

[13] Limbrock GJ, Fischer-Brandies H, Avalle C. Castillo-Morales' orofacial therapy: treatment of 67 children with Down syndrome. Dev Med Child Neurol.; 33(4):296–303

[14] Inga CJ, Reddy AK, Richardson SA, Sanders B. Appliance for chronic drooling in cerebral palsy patients. Pediatr Dent.; 23 (3):241–242

[15] Wong V, Sun JG, Wong W. Traditional Chinese medicine (tongue acupuncture) in children with drooling problems. Pediatr Neurol.; 25(1):47–54

[16] Mier RJ, Bachrach SJ, Lakin RC, Barker T, Childs J, Moran M. Treatment of sialorrhea with glycopyrrolate: a double-blind, dose-ranging study. Arch Pediatr Adolesc Med.; 154(12): 1214–1218

[17] Talmi YP, Finkelstein Y, Zohar Y. Reduction of salivary flow with transdermal scopolamine: a four-year experience. Otolaryngol Head Neck Surg.; 103(4):615–618

[18] Dashtipour K, Bhidayasiri R, Chen JJ, Jabbari B, Lew M, Torres-Russotto D. RimabotulinumtoxinB in sialorrhea: systematic review of clinical trials. J Clin Mov Disord.; 4:9

[19] Petracca M, Guidubaldi A, Ricciardi L, et al. Botulinum Toxin A and B in sialorrhea: long-term data and literature overview. Toxicon.; 107 Pt A:129–140

[20] Lim YC, Choi EC. Treatment of an acute salivary fistula after parotid surgery: botulinum toxin type A injection as primary treatment. Eur Arch Otorhinolaryngol.; 265(2):243–245

[21] Laskawi R, Winterhoff J, Köhler S, Kottwitz L, Matthias C. Botulinum toxin treatment of salivary fistulas following parotidectomy: follow-up results. Oral Maxillofac Surg.; 17(4): 281–285

[22] Tiigimäe-Saar J, Taba P, Tamme T. Does Botulinum neurotoxin type A treatment for sialorrhea change oral health? Clin Oral Investig.; 21(3):795–800

[23] Marina MB, Sani A, Hamzaini AH, Hamidon BB. Ultrasound-guided botulinum toxin A injection: an alternative treatment for dribbling. J Laryngol Otol.; 122(6):609–614

[24] Borg M, Hirst F. The role of radiation therapy in the management of sialorrhea. Int J Radiat Oncol Biol Phys.; 41 (5):1113–1119

[25] Frederick FJ, Stewart IF. Effectiveness of transtympanic neurectomy in management of sialorrhea occurring in mentally retarded patients. J Otolaryngol.; 11(4):289–292

[26] O'Neil LM, Palme CE, Riffat F, Mahant N. Botulinum toxin for the management of Sjögren syndrome-associated recurrent parotitis. J Oral Maxillofac Surg.; 74(12):2428–2430

[27] Daniel SJ, Diamond M. Botulinum toxin injection: a novel treatment for recurrent cystic parotitis Sjögren syndrome. Otolaryngol Head Neck Surg.; 145(1):180–181

[28] Kruegel J, Winterhoff J, Koehler S, Matthes P, Laskawi R. Botulinum toxin: a noninvasive option for the symptomatic treatment of salivary gland stenosis - a case report. Head Neck.; 32(7):959–963

20

Botulinum Neurotoxin for Radiation-Induced Spasm and Pain

Diana N. Kirke, Brian E. Benson, and Tanya K. Meyer

Summary

Botulinum neurotoxin (BoNT) can be applied to the treatment of the sequelae resulting from radiation therapy for head and neck cancer (HNC). The term "radiation fibrosis syndrome" (RFS) encompasses these sequelae and includes muscle spasm, both cervical dystonia and trismus, and neuropathic pain which includes trigeminal neuralgia, cervical plexus neuralgia, and migraine. The importance of treating HNC patients lies in the fact that almost half continue to suffer from chronic pain following the completion of treatment and are thus at risk of opioid misuse. With long-term survival now a possibility, this can indeed impact upon quality of life. This chapter discusses the appropriate workup required and the injection technique as they relate to radiated HNC patients.

Keywords: botulinum neurotoxin, head and neck, pain, radiation, spasm

20.1 Introduction

The use of botulinum neurotoxin (BoNT) for head and neck disorders can also be extended to the sequelae resulting from the treatment for head and neck cancer (HNC). These complications include chronic and neuropathic pain following neck dissection, muscle spasms after radiation therapy, and radiation-induced trismus and fibrosis.[1] In fact, pain affects 45% of patients in the years following treatment, with a quarter of those patients describing severe pain.[2] With long-term survival becoming more common, the pain impacts quality of life (QOL) and can result in major depression, anxiety, and reduced recreation.[2,3] This is concerning because this may lead to the use of opioid-containing medications that may place one at the risk of misuse. Patients with a HNC diagnosis are more likely to be prescribed opioids, as opposed to those with other cancer diagnoses such as lung cancer and colon cancer.[4] While the analgesic effects of BoNT are still unclear, there is evidence to suggest that its use can play an important role in helping to mitigate the physical sequelae following treatment for HNC.[1,5,6,7,8] Furthermore, the use of BoNT as an adjunctive treatment was recently recommended in the Head and Neck Cancer Survivorship Guidelines for both cervical dystonia (CD) and the pain associated with trismus.[3]

Radiation fibrosis syndrome (RFS) is a term that has been used to describe the complications following radiation therapy and defines complications into two general categories, including muscle spasm and neuropathic pain. Muscle spasm incorporates CD and trismus, while neuropathic pain incorporates trigeminal neuralgia, cervical plexus neuralgia, and migraine.[1] Using RFS as a framework, this chapter will discuss each of the following conditions in turn, referencing back to previous chapters, as well as highlighting the important issues as they relate to the HNC patient[1]:

- Muscle spasm:
  - Cervical dystonia.
  - Trismus.
- Neuropathic pain:
  - Trigeminal neuralgia.
  - Cervical plexus neuralgia.
  - Migraine.

20.2 Workup

The patient should have a complete history and examination performed by their treating physician/surgeon in order to rule out the possibility that their symptoms could be attributed to a recurrent or new malignancy. If there is a suspicion, then an appropriate evaluation including imaging of the area should be undertaken. If there is no recurrent or new malignancy and the patient has failed treatment with standard conservative and medical management, then they can be considered a candidate for BoNT injection into the affected areas. Conservative management may include physical therapy for myofascial release, range of movement training, and lymphedema management. Medical management may include the use of analgesics such as acetaminophen, ibuprofen, opioids, topical lidocaine, as well as nerve stabilizing agents such as gabapentin and amitriptyline. How many medical treatments the patient must fail prior to starting treatment with BoNT is unknown, but one study does suggest a failure of at least

two.[5] Important metrics to consider pre- and postinjection include a visual analog scale (VAS) for pain and the QOL scale that is most pertinent to the patient.

20.3 Anatomy and Technique

The anatomy and injection technique have been described in Chapter 7 (cervical dystonia), Chapter 12 (temporomandibular disorders), Chapter 14 (migraine), and Chapter 16 (trigeminal neuralgia). There are, however, some important considerations as they relate to HNC patients, which will be discussed here as they relate to the RFS framework. The dosages for the muscles injected are summarized in ▶ Fig. 20.1.

20.3.1 Muscle Spasm

Cervical Dystonia

The muscle spasm of the neck seen in the irradiated HNC patient is not a dystonia by the classical definition, but certainly it is related to a sustained fixation of the cervical muscles leading to abnormal posturing of the neck, head, and shoulder. This is due to radiation fibrosis of the cervical musculature, which in turn results in involuntary spasm with or without myofascial pain. The current Head and Neck Cancer Survivorship guidelines recommend referral for BoNT-A injections if such findings are found on examination.[3] The muscles that can be treated are those that generally cause laterocollis and include the ipsilateral sternocleidomastoid (SCM), splenius capitis, scalene complex, levator scapulae, and trapezius; see ▶ Table 7.1 and ▶ Fig. 7.1 in Chapter 7.

If a covering flap has been used (e.g., pectoralis major myocutaneous flap), then this too can be affected.[9] Like CD there is

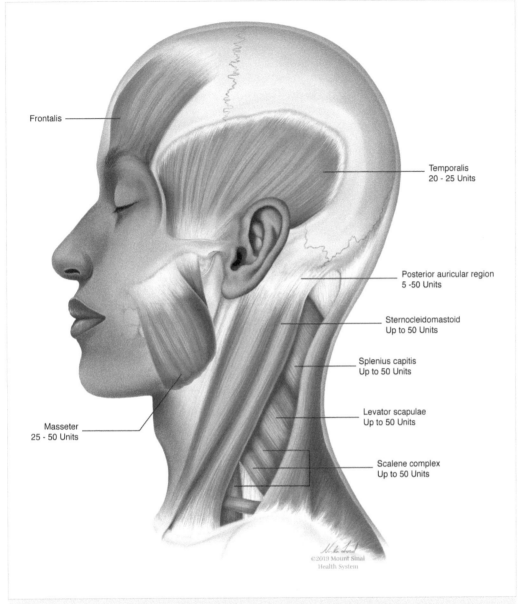

Fig. 20.1 Possible sites requiring botulinum neurotoxin (BoNT) injection in the radiated head and neck cancer patient, with associated dosages of BoNT-A outlined. (Printed with permission from Mount Sinai Health System.)

variation in the muscles injected; however, the injection should be performed at the site of peak contracture which can be assessed by palpating a firm cord in the neck (▶ Video 20.1).[9] There is also variation in dosages used, with one study reporting an average of 22 U of BoNT-A to each muscle in order to avoid impairment of swallowing function, yet another used doses in the magnitude normally used to treat CD (200–300 U of BoNT-A), with no dose reductions required.[6,8]

Trismus

Trismus can occur in up to 38% of individuals postradiation therapy, and is quantitatively defined as a ≤ 35 mm maximal interincisal distance.[3] Trismus develops as a result of radiation fibrosis in the masticator muscles; is often associated with pain; and can impact eating, speaking, and the maintenance of oral hygiene.[7] In the only study thus far to measure interincisal distance pre- and post-BoNT injection, trismus did not improve with bilateral injection of the masseters, but pain did.[7] Therefore, the use of BoNT-A is considered an adjunctive treatment as supported by the Head and Neck Cancer Survivorship guidelines.[3] As with injection of the masseters for other temporomandibular joint disorders, the starting dose should be 25 U and not exceed 50 U BoNT-A per masseter.[6]

20.3.2 Neuropathic Pain

Trigeminal Neuralgia

This can also occur in the irradiated HNC patient with the symptoms as described in Chapter 16. Dosages in the range of 70 to 200 U of BoNT-A have been reported in this subset of patients.[1]

Cervical Plexus Neuralgia

Neuropathic pain sites in the HNC patient are generally in the distribution of the cervical plexus.[10] This type of pain can be described as a burning or shooting pain and/or allodynia. Unlike the widespread use of BoNT in neck contracture, analgesia in this case can generally be obtained by injecting the site of the pain.[9]

Migraine

This can also occur in the irradiated HNC patient with the symptoms as described in Chapter 14. Dosages in the range of 100 U of BoNT-A have been reported in this subset of patients.[1]

20.4 Follow-up

Patients should follow up at 2 weeks postinjection to assess response. If response is suboptimal, then additional injections can be administered using the same technique, while if the response is otherwise satisfactory then patients can follow up on an as-needed basis.

20.5 Complications and Pitfalls

The complications relating to these injection techniques have been described in Chapter 7 (cervical dystonia), Chapter 12 (temporomandibular disorders), Chapter 14 (migraine), and Chapter 16 (trigeminal neuralgia). There are, however, some pertinent considerations as they relate to HNC patients. These include the possibility of the temporary worsening of dysphagia and dry mouth, which is already a concern in such patients. While transient and generally lasting no longer than 2 weeks, these complications can be tempered with a dose reduction, particularly when injecting the anterior neck, as well as preferentially injecting more superiorly in order to keep the diffusion of BoNT away from the pharyngeal musculature.[1]

20.6 Key Points/Pearls

- Botulinum neurotoxin can be used to treat the early and late sequelae following both surgical treatment and chemoradiation for head and neck cancer.

- Syndromes that it can address broadly include muscle spasms and neuropathic pain.
  - Muscle spasms include cervical dystonia and trismus.
  - Neuropathic pain includes trigeminal neuralgia, cervical plexus neuralgia, and migraine.

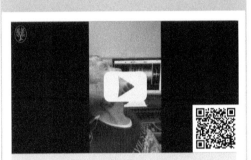

Video 20.1 Cervical dystonia. This patient has painful spasms of bilateral sternocleidomastoid (SCM) musculature following radiation treatment for laryngeal cancer. He receives EMG-guided injections of 25 units into bilateral SCM (right SCM shown in the video), the muscle activity of which is heard when the patient pushes against the injector's contralateral hand. [0:45]

References

[1] Stubblefield MD, Levine A, Custodio CM, Fitzpatrick T. The role of botulinum toxin type A in the radiation fibrosis syndrome: a preliminary report. Arch Phys Med Rehabil.; 89(3): 417–421

[2] Cramer JD, Johnson JT, Nilsen ML. Pain in head and neck cancer survivors: prevalence, predictors, and quality-of-life impact. Otolaryngol Head Neck Surg.; 159(5):853–858

[3] Cohen EEW, LaMonte SJ, Erb NL, Beckman KL, Sadeghi N, Hutcheson KA, et al. American Cancer Society Head and Neck Cancer Survivorship Care Guideline. CA Cancer J Clin.; 66(3): 203–39

[4] Sethi RKV, Panth N, Puram SV, Varvares MA. Opioid prescription patterns among patients with head and neck cancer. JAMA Otolaryngol Head Neck Surg.; 144(4):382–383

[5] Rostami R, Mittal SO, Radmand R, Jabbari B. Incobotulinum toxin-A improves post-surgical and post-radiation pain in cancer patients. Toxins (Basel).; 8(1):22–28

[6] Mittal S, Machado DG, Jabbari B. OnabotulinumtoxinA for treatment of focal cancer pain after surgery and/or radiation. Pain Med.; 13(8):1029–1033

[7] Hartl DM, Cohen M, Juliéron M, Marandas P, Janot F, Bourhis J. Botulinum toxin for radiation-induced facial pain and trismus. Otolaryngol Head Neck Surg.; 138(4):459–463

[8] Van Daele DJ, Finnegan EM, Rodnitzky RL, Zhen W, McCulloch TM, Hoffman HT. Head and neck muscle spasm after radiotherapy: management with botulinum toxin A injection. Arch Otolaryngol Head Neck Surg.; 128(8):956–959

[9] Bach CA, Wagner I, Lachiver X, Baujat B, Chabolle F. Botulinum toxin in the treatment of post-radiosurgical neck contracture in head and neck cancer: a novel approach. Eur Ann Otorhinolaryngol Head Neck dis.; 129(1):6–10

[10] Wittekindt C, Liu W-C, Preuss SF, Guntinas-Lichius O. Botulinum toxin A for neuropathic pain after neck dissection: a dose-finding study. Laryngoscope.; 116(7):1168–1171

Index